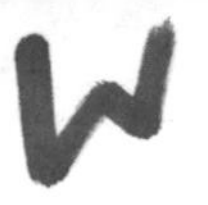

Overcoming Common Problems

The Fertility Handbook

Medical and self-help treatments to help you conceive

DR PHILIPPA KAYE

sheldon PRESS

First published in Great Britain in 2007

Sheldon Press
36 Causton Street
London SW1P 4ST

The author and publisher have made every effort to ensure that the external website and email addresses included in this book are correct and up to date at the time of going to press. The author and publisher are not responsible for the content, quality or continuing accessibility of the sites.

British Library Cataloguing-in-Publication Data
A catalogue record for this book is available from the British Library

ISBN 978–1–84709–016–4

1 3 5 7 9 10 8 6 4 2

Typeset by Fakenham Photosetting Ltd, Fakenham, Norfolk
Printed in Great Britain by Ashford Colour Press

Produced on paper from sustainable forests

Contents

Introduction

When I started writing this book I asked some children what they wanted to be when they grew up. Among the responses of fireman, ballerina, footballer, popstar and superhero there were some more traditional answers:

> I will get married and go to work to get money for my wife and all the children. I have to get money to look after them. (Robbie, 5)
>
> I want to be a mummy. Girls can grow babies in their tummies, I want a baby in my tummy. (Priya, 5)
>
> I am going to have 17 children. (Danny, 4)

It seems that even from a very early age children are aware of their roles in society and of the need to reproduce. Perhaps it is a basic animal need, like the need to eat or drink, perhaps it is a need to nurture, a need to create or a need to pass something of yourself on. I have even heard having children described as the only true path to immortality, that in your children and children's children, you can live for ever.

The World Health Organization defines health as: 'A state of complete physical, mental and social well being and not merely the absence of disease or infirmity.' This means that health is not simply about not having an illness but about being happy in all aspects of your life. The definition has been criticized as being impossible to obtain for everyone all of the time. However, it does show that even if you are well, have everything you need materially, have a happy relationship, if there is something missing, if you are not entirely content, then you could be considered unhealthy. For many people, the thing that is missing is a child.

The term infertility means that you are absolutely unable to conceive. The more common situation is subfertility – you can conceive, but may need a little help to do so. Subfertility is defined as not conceiving after a year of unprotected regular sexual intercourse. Subfertility can be primary or secondary: primary if you have never been pregnant and secondary if you have had previous pregnancies (though these could have resulted in miscarriages or terminations). Many people have told me they feel guilty for wanting further children when they already have a child, and others have none. Many of the emotions described in this book are the same whether you have no children or many. If you want a child and you are having difficulty in conceiving, you may experience similar emotions.

A common misconception is that if you are struggling to conceive, you are alone. Suddenly, everyone you know has children, or you walk down the street and notice all the pregnant women, or those with pushchairs. About 15 per cent of couples – about one in six – are affected, so it is more common than you probably think. It is reassuring to note that of this 15 per cent, about half will conceive naturally.

There is also a belief that subfertility is increasing. This may be related to the fact that many women delay starting a family. Or perhaps, as there are now more treatments available and less stigma attached to subfertility, more couples are presenting for help. Subfertility is common, controversial and a current 'hot topic'. While writing this book, in the first two months, I collected over two large files of newspaper and magazine cuttings about fertility, subfertility and its treatment. What you should do, what you shouldn't do, the latest wonder drug, postcode lottery, etc. There are a multitude of documentaries and dramas based around the topic on television, the radio and in the cinema. The internet is full of websites about the topic. Quite simply, you cannot get away from it, and we are assaulted with information, much of it contradictory and confusing.

This book aims to guide you through the process of diagnosing and treating any problems you may be having getting pregnant. I hope to guide you from when to go to the doctor, how to help yourself, how to get treatment and to tell you what happens at each appointment, investigation and treatment. It is well known that people forget what the doctor tells them, and in my experience no matter how many times you explain something verbally, people absorb information better if they are also given written explanations. The book aims to take away some of the fear around subfertility by explaining stage by stage what may happen, and some of the emotions that may arise.

Although many of the cases described in the book have happy endings, I have tried to include both positive and negative stories as at some point you may feel the same way as those whose stories are told. Simply identifying the emotion, and recognizing that you are not the only person ever to feel that way, may help you.

Medicine, science and technology are fast-changing. The guidelines doctors use change when new research and studies are published; investigation and treatment options change as new technologies are discovered. As medicine changes, so does the law. The information in this book is correct at the time of writing, and your doctor should inform you of any new research and treatments. No book, or the internet, can ever replace a one-to-one medical consultation which involves your doctor taking a history, examining you, and tailoring any investigations and treatments specifically to you.

Finally, a common belief appears to be that if you are having difficulties in getting pregnant you are less of a woman or man, a failure in your sexual role. Remember, there is a difference between virility and fertility, femininity and fecundity. You are as much of a man or woman as the next person, perhaps more so as you are stepping up and saying you want help and will do whatever it takes to get what you need. Many people say they feel a failure, that they cannot do the most natural thing in the world, and that they feel guilty for inflicting this process on their partner (ignoring the fact that in many cases both partners have factors). Although I can understand why you may feel that way and can appreciate that I may feel the same in a similar situation, I would like to tell you I think that you could not be further from the truth. You are not failures, but some of the strongest, most courageous and resilient people. People who admit to themselves that there is a problem and then set about finding a strategy to overcome it, who put themselves through thick and thin to achieve their end. I wish you all the best of luck.

1

The process of conception

Conception, the process in which an egg and sperm fuse together, is the start of any pregnancy. Understanding conception and some of the medical terms used to describe it will hopefully help you get the most out of this book, and from any medical consultation, procedure or treatment that you may undergo. Different tests and treatments are used depending on the cause of the problems, so a basic understanding of the natural process and where, if at all, your difficulty lies, will help you make sense of the sometimes stressful times which may follow.

In order to become pregnant the following conditions have to be met:

- an egg must be produced by the woman;
- sperm must be produced by the man and released into the woman;
- the sperm must reach the egg and join with it – fertilization;
- the fertilized egg must implant in the womb of the woman.

The female menstrual cycle

The menstrual cycle is the monthly sequence of hormonal changes that lead to the production of an egg. These hormones also lead to changes in the womb to prepare it for implantation if an egg were to be fertilized. If an egg is not fertilized, menstruation, your period, will follow.

A woman is born with all her eggs – many hundreds of thousands – in an immature state. Not all will develop into mature eggs; many will be absorbed by the body. Only about 400 are released in all the menstrual cycles in your entire life. You cannot produce any new eggs; each month when an egg is released at ovulation, it is one of the eggs that you already have, which has matured.

There are three levels of hormonal control, which interact with each other to control the menstrual cycle:

- Brain – an area of the brain called the hypothalamus secretes a hormone called gonadotrophin releasing hormone (GnRH).
- Brain – the pituitary gland releases two hormones in response to

GnRH. These hormones are called gonadotrophins; they are follicle-stimulating hormone (FSH) and luteinizing hormone (LH).
- Ovaries – produce two hormones, oestrogen and progesterone in response to the production of FSH and LH.

The length of the menstrual cycle is variable. Only one in ten women have a 28-day cycle, and it is normal for your cycle to be between 21 to 35 days, though some women have even longer or shorter cycles. The explanation below is calculated for a 28-day cycle. If your cycle is longer or shorter than this, each stage of the cycle will be longer or shorter as appropriate.

Days 1–5 menstruation: Day 1 of your menstrual cycle is the first day of your period, which lasts an average of five days. The 'blood' of your period is a combination of shedding the thick lining of the womb (endometrium) and blood.

Days 5–13 follicular/proliferative phase: The hypothalamus starts releasing GnRH. This acts on the pituitary to stimulate the release of FSH and LH. These hormones then act on the ovary to stimulate the growth of eggs within fluid-filled sacs called follicles.

Days 8–10: About 20 follicles grow but one follicle then grows larger than the others, and will be the follicle to produce an egg. The growing follicles produce oestrogen which causes the lining of the womb to become thick in readiness for a fertilized egg.

Day 14 ovulation: As the level of oestrogen produced by the follicles peaks, it affects the pituitary gland, causing a short, sharp rise in the secretion of LH. The peak of LH secretion causes ovulation to occur about 16–32 hours later – an egg pops out of the most mature follicle in the ovary and is released. The released egg is picked up by the fimbria and is transported into the fallopian tube.

There is also a peak of oestrogen at this point. The other follicles from which eggs have not been released overripen and break down. The egg then travels down the fallopian tube into the uterus (womb), a journey that takes on average five days.

Days 14–28 luteal/secretory phase: The follicle that produced the egg is now an empty shell, called the corpus luteum, which produces some oestrogen but relatively more of the other ovarian hormone, progesterone. As this phase continues, more and more progesterone is produced. Levels of progesterone peak around day 21 of the cycle.

Progesterone acts on the now thickened lining of the womb to prepare it for implantation. The glands in the lining secrete a

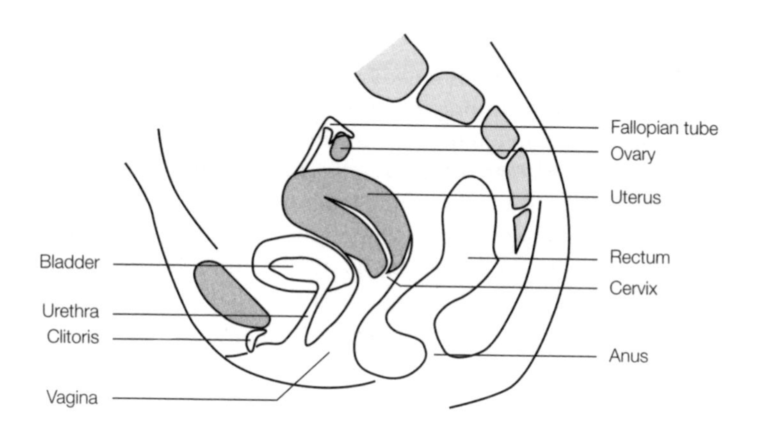

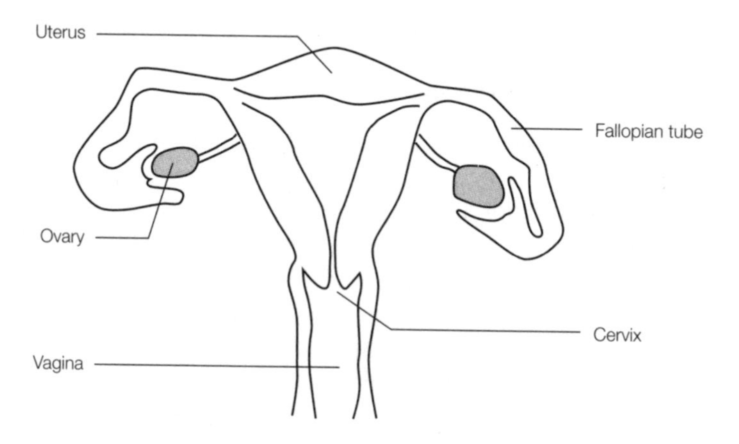

Figure 1 The anatomy of the female reproductive system

substance to help feed a fertilized egg for a few days until the placenta is formed. This secretion happens even if there is no fertilized egg. The corpus luteum survives for about 14 days and if an egg is not fertilized, it breaks down, causing levels of both oestrogen and progesterone to fall.

The lining of the womb is reliant on oestrogen and progesterone, so as the levels of these hormones fall, the blood supply to the lining is cut off. Without the oxygen and nutrients supplied by the blood the tissue breaks down and menstruation occurs. The cycle then restarts as the falling levels of hormones act on the brain to release pulses of GnRH to restart the cycle. If, however, implantation of an embryo has occurred the hormone levels will remain high and the lining of the womb will not be shed – the reason why you don't get periods in pregnancy.

So, hopefully at approximately day 14 an egg is released from its follicle in the ovary into the fallopian tube. Now we need some sperm.

Spermatogenesis

Spermatogenesis means the production of sperm. Unlike women, who are born with all their eggs, men don't start producing sperm until puberty but then go on producing new sperm for the rest of their lives.

As in the menstrual cycle in women there are three levels of hormonal control, which all interact to result in spermatogenesis, a process which takes approximately 70 days:

- Brain – the hypothalamus secretes gonadotrophin releasing hormone (GnRH).
- Brain – the anterior pituitary gland releases follicle-stimulating hormone (FSH) and luteinizing hormone (LH) in response to GnRH.
- Testes – produce the hormones testosterone and oestrogen.

First, as with women, the hypothalamus secretes GnRH which in turn stimulates the anterior pituitary gland to secrete FSH and LH. LH acts on the testes to produce testosterone, FSH acts on cells involved in the making and transport of sperm. The testosterone produced acts on the brain to restart the cycle.

The hormones make immature sperm cells multiply and then undergo a process to shape the sperm. Sperm have large heads containing genetic material and long tails enabling them to move. The sperm are released into the seminiferous tubules to travel to the epididymis, where they are stored for approximately two weeks in

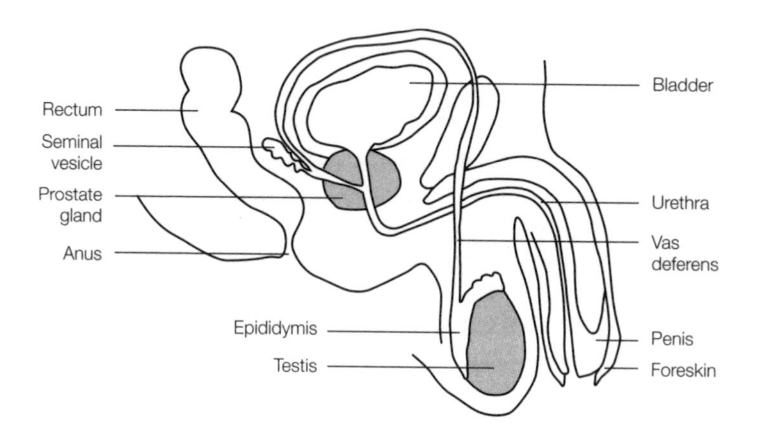

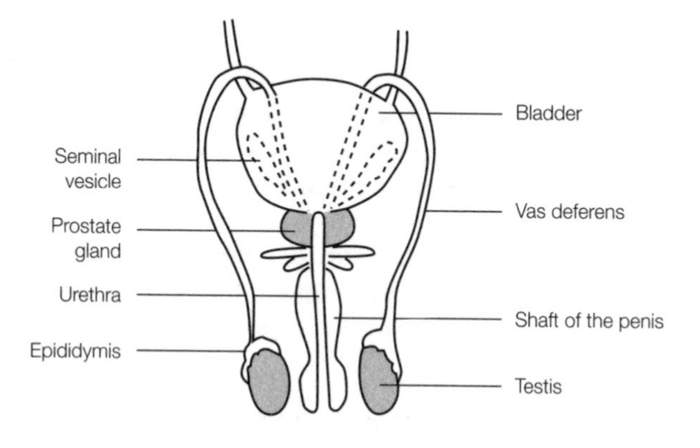

Figure 2 The anatomy of the male reproductive system

order to become capable of fertilizing an egg. Sperm travel from the epididymis to the penis via a tube called the vas deferens. On male ejaculation, a white fluid called semen is released. Between 40 and 600 million sperm are released in the semen, along with other fluids.

So, we now have an egg and some sperm…

Fertilization

Fertilization is the process by which a sperm and an egg fuse together. Humans have 46 chromosomes in every cell that contain their genetic makeup. Eggs and sperm each carry 23 chromosomes. Once they join they become a cell with a complete set of 46 chromosomes that eventually form a baby.

During sexual intercourse, the semen, containing the sperm, is deposited at the neck of the womb, or cervix. The vagina is an acidic environment, hostile to sperm, so the semen clumps together to protect the sperm against the acid. Of the millions of sperm that are released, only a small percentage enter the uterus via the cervix and only the strongest survive to potentially meet an egg.

If sex occurs around the time of ovulation, the uterus has already been primed for the sperm by oestrogen. Oestrogen also helps prepare the sperm for fertilization by making their tails whip back and forth to move them along. If ovulation has occurred the sperm may meet an egg in the tubes. An egg needs to be fertilized within approximately 24 hours of ovulation, otherwise it will begin to break down. Sperm, however, may survive for a few days while waiting to meet an egg.

A single sperm enters an egg and fertilizes it. At this point, the fertilized egg is called the 'zygote'. The male and female chromosomes join together and the cell replicates and divides. It then takes approximately three to four days for the zygote to travel through the fallopian tube into the womb, from which point it is called the 'blastocyst'.

Implantation

Implantation is when the blastocyst inserts itself into the lining of the uterus. The blastocyst generally remains in the womb for one to three days before implantation occurs, approximately five to seven days after ovulation. Once implanted the cells replicate to form the placenta, membranes and embryo. The term embryo is used to describe the early stage of development, up to eight weeks of gestation, and after this it is called the foetus.

As described above there are four conditions that need to be met in order for pregnancy to occur: ovulation, spermatogenesis, fertilization and implantation. If there is a problem in any of these areas pregnancy may not occur without help.

What are the odds of getting pregnant?

As complex as the process of conception is, for an average couple, the odds of conceiving within any particular menstrual cycle each month are between 20 and 25 per cent, that is one in four or five. The odds remain the same for each cycle – that is, each month you have a 20–25 per cent chance. Sometimes conception takes a long time, even if there are no problems. About 80 per cent of women will fall pregnant within a year of regular unprotected sexual intercourse. This increases to approximately 90 per cent, i.e. nine out of ten women, after two years of regular unprotected sex.

When to ask for help from the doctor

The desire to have a baby can be so strong that not getting pregnant in the first month can be hugely upsetting and frustrating. However, it is important to remember that only one in five women get pregnant in the first month of trying.

Subfertility is defined as a failure to conceive after one year of regular unprotected sexual intercourse. Therefore, if you have not conceived after a year it is reasonable to make an appointment with your GP to discuss the situation and to be assessed for further investigations and treatment. Admitting it is time to see a doctor can be hard…

> Months passed, each with its hopeful anxiety followed by crushing disappointment. As time went on I began to get more and more worried that something was wrong but kept my feelings to myself, and kept on trying. Time passed and my partner suggested to me that we went to see our doctor; the strength of my reaction surprised even myself. I was furious with him for suggesting it. I realize now that my anger was a cover for my real emotions – upset, but most of all scared, no … terrified. Going to the doctor meant that I had to admit to myself that there may be a problem, that I may not be able to get pregnant, that I may need some help. I wasn't sure that I was ready to face that. (Tara, 31)

Many couples find that waiting for a year feels like an eternity. There are various techniques and lifestyle modifications that you can use to increase your chances of getting pregnant (see Chapter 3, How to increase your fertility). If you feel that the wait is making you so stressed and anxious that it is decreasing your fertility, then making an appointment to see your doctor is not unreasonable. It may be that your doctor may be able to reassure you or advise you on the techniques described in Chapter 3.

For some people, it is advisable to seek medical advice earlier than the recommended year:

Women

- Aged over 35 years
- Not having periods at all (amenorrhoea)
- Having periods infrequently (oligomenorrhoea)
- Previous ectopic pregnancy (pregnancy outside the womb)
- Previous surgery to the fallopian tubes or in the pelvis
- Known disease in the fallopian tubes
- History of pelvic inflammatory disease or sexually transmitted infections
- Large fibroids

Men

- History of sexually transmitted disease
- Previous surgery to the genitals, pelvis or groin region
- History of undescended testicles (cryptorchidism) and/or the operation to pull undescended testicles into the scrotum (orchidopexy)
- History of chemotherapy
- History of radiotherapy
- Presence of a varicocele – a dilation of the veins within the testicles

If you or your partner have, or have had, any of the above conditions, do visit your doctor earlier than one year, perhaps after six months. He or she may advise waiting for spontaneous conception, but it may also be appropriate to carry out investigations at an earlier stage.

2

Starting your journey

Before you start your journey to conceiving a baby and pregnancy, and during the process, it is important you are aware of some of the issues that may arise. It is impossible to fully prepare yourself for every eventuality but by talking over some of the potential situations with your partner or a third party, you can prepare yourself, and consider some of the more difficult subjects. Of course, no one can predict what will happen; it may be that you conceive naturally or with minimal input, or you may need more treatment. You cannot predict how you will feel at each stage but thinking about some of the issues that may arise is invaluable. Some topics are practical and others emotional and some questions may as yet be unanswerable.

Some topics and questions to discuss

The following list, although long, is not exhaustive. More issues may arise, while some of the situations may not be relevant in your case. There are no right or wrong answers to these questions; just your emotions and how you feel about the topics raised. Simply talking around some of these topics may help you along this journey.

- Who will attend each appointment? Will you both attend every appointment, blood test, investigation and procedure?
- Can you both afford to attend every appointment in terms of time away from work?
- Where do you feel you need most support – for example, could you cope with a blood test alone or are you needle phobic?
- Would you like time to talk to your doctor alone?
- Would you like a third party such as a friend or other family member to attend some appointments?
- How far away is the clinic? How will you get there? How much will travel/parking cost?
- Will you be allowed to take time off work to attend appointments?
- What are you prepared, and not prepared, to do in terms of investigations and treatment?

- Are you prepared to continue if the NHS cannot start or continue to fund your treatment?
- Are you prepared for the physical effects of treatment: including side effects of drugs such as mood swings?
- Are you aware of the possibility of failure at the many steps along the way? How do you think you will feel, how will you support each other?
- If you do get pregnant, are you aware of the possibility of miscarriage? How do you think you would cope with it?
- How do you feel about having twins or triplets, remembering the risks involved to both mother and children? Could you physically/emotionally/financially cope with a multiple birth?
- If you freeze embryos, what will happen to them if you and your partner were to split up?
- How will you try to support and talk to the other person? How will you still try to make time for 'us'? Would counselling help, either separately or together?
- How many times can you afford to try – physically/emotionally/financially? Are you prepared to go into debt or to remortgage in order to fund treatment? Or to enter an egg sharing scheme in order to cover costs?
- Would you consider using donor eggs or sperm or embryos? How would you feel about a child that is not genetically yours?
- Would you consider surrogacy, fostering or adoption?
- Who of your family, friends, work colleagues or bosses do you tell? Does your partner mind you discussing it?
- Is one of you a pessimist or an optimist? How does that make the other partner feel?
- If you are going through this procedure alone, for example using donor sperm, will you pick one person to be your companion through investigations, or many?
- How much will you tell your child about how he or she was conceived?

The first appointment – what happens?

For most people, your GP will be your first port of call – as already said, this is often a difficult step.

> Convincing my partner to go to our GP was probably the hardest part of the process. He said there was no way he would talk about sex with a doctor, that it was private. He got angry too, until he

> realized how much each month of emptiness meant to him, as well as me, then it was him that dragged me! (Elle, 31)
>
> I went to my local surgery three times: the first time I said I had a cold, the second time I saw a different doctor, I nearly told her but then couldn't so I asked her for some hayfever tablets. It was November so she wouldn't give them to me, I knew she knew there was something else as she kept asking, but I couldn't tell her. The third time I plucked up the courage to tell her we were trying, and failing, to have a baby. (Jenny, 34)
>
> I went to my GP because we had been trying for nine months. Having looked it up online I thought he would send me away. That was what I wanted really, a good doctor whom I trusted to reassure me, tell me it was all going to be okay. But he didn't. He asked me loads of questions, and because I had had an ectopic pregnancy years back, he referred me to a gynaecologist. It was only then that I really started panicking; after all, if the doctor was concerned, then something was really up, it was then that the fear kicked in. (Sarah, 32)

The first appointment generally involves talking and an examination. Many GPs only have very short appointment slots to see patients. They may ask you to come back another time so they can book you a longer slot. They will ask you questions such as:

- How long have you been trying for a baby?
- How often are you having unprotected sex?
- Do you take any medication?
- Do you have any other children?
- How long is your menstrual cycle?
- Have you ever had an ectopic pregnancy?
- Have you had any previous sexually transmitted diseases?
- Have you had any previous surgery or illness?

These questions form what doctors call the patient's 'history'. By asking them, doctors are trying to find out as much as they can about the problem and any factors in your past that may be contributing to your subfertility. Your GP will also need to ask your partner questions, and you may have your appointments together or separately.

Your doctor may simply reassure you and give you advice on increasing your chances of becoming pregnant, such as described in Chapter 3, How to increase your fertility. For example, if as a couple you have no risk factors for subfertility and have been having regular unprotected sex for six months, your doctor may reassure you but ask you to come back if you have not conceived after a year of unprotected sex.

> I was so relieved when my doctor told me to go away and keep trying. I had got so caught up in the excitement of getting pregnant that after five months of trying I was absolutely gutted that nothing was happening and was getting a bit stressed about it. She told me that I was normal and to keep trying – the relief of being told that not being pregnant after five months was not abnormal! Three months later, she was right and I was pregnant. (Karen, 31)

If your GP agrees with you that there may be a problem with your fertility, he or she can refer you to a gynaecologist, andrologist or fertility centre. The referral can be made under the NHS or privately.

Your doctor may also examine you both. These examinations are likely to be repeated by hospital doctors.

Women

- Speculum examination – as in a smear test, the walls of the vagina are pushed back with an instrument called a speculum, so the cervix can be seen. This examination is uncomfortable; however, the more relaxed you are the easier and less uncomfortable it is, so do try to relax and focus on your breathing. The examination lasts a few minutes at most. Swabs can be taken at this point to rule out infection. If you are over 25 and have not had a smear in the last three years a cervical smear could also be taken during the speculum examination.
- Vaginal examination – the doctor inserts two fingers into the vagina while their other hand gently presses on your lower tummy. They are feeling for the cervix and aim to feel the uterus and ovaries moving between their hands. Masses such as fibroids or cysts may be felt in this way.

If you are being examined by a male doctor there will always be a female chaperone present in the room. Some female doctors will always have a chaperone, others will give you the choice of whether you want a chaperone.

Men

The genitalia will be examined, for example to check testicular size or feel for a varicocele.

Initial tests

While you wait for your hospital appointment, there are various tests your GP can organize so that by the time you get to see the fertility doctors they already have the results. (For more information on the tests themselves, see Chapter 6, Diagnostic tests.)

In women, blood tests may check:

- levels of FSH, LH and oestrogen, on day 2 to 3 of your menstrual cycle;
- progesterone levels to check if you have ovulated on day 21, or seven days before your period is due;
- thyroid function and level of prolactin;
- rubella immunity.

An ultrasound scan may also be arranged to check the structure of your reproductive organs.

In men, semen analysis may be arranged.

Your GP is important. Not only does he or she look after your general health, arrange tests or refer you, but they can also offer counselling, or simply be another person to talk to. He or she may explain how the funding of treatment works, or put you in touch with a support group. Whatever stage of treatment you are at, remember that your GP is there as someone to talk to and ask advice from.

Once at the gynaecologist or fertility centre, the first appointment, and indeed a large percentage of appointments will involve taking a history and talking. Other tests can be organized – see Chapter 6, Diagnostic tests.

Get the most from your appointments

For every appointment, be it at the GP, hospital or a fertility clinic:

- Make a list of questions beforehand that you wish to ask the doctor.
- If you wish to be seen by a female doctor, please ring or write to the clinic first.
- All male doctors will be chaperoned during any examinations. If you would like a female doctor, or to have a chaperone during an examination, please ask.
- If possible, take somebody with you. It is well known that most people forget most of what the doctor says to them; somebody else can help you absorb the information. The support of a second person can also be useful.

- Ask if there is any written information you can have to read later.
- It is all right to ask doctors to repeat themselves, or to answer questions.
- Ask if it is possible to contact someone if you have further questions, and how – by letter, phone, email or make another appointment. Ask if there is an emergency contact number.
- When discussing investigations and treatments you should be told about alternatives and why the doctor feels a particular option is best for you. You should be told about the potential benefits and risks such as side effects. If not, ask!
- If you are also taking complementary medicines, please inform your doctor.

Choosing a clinic and getting treatment

You can see a fertility specialist under the NHS or privately. In both situations your first port of call is your GP, who will refer you if appropriate.

National Health Service

In the NHS, the 'choose and book' system allows you to choose from a limited number of local hospitals and clinics for your first appointment. You should be given at least four choices and will also be able to book the most convenient date and time. You can research your options using the questions described below under 'Other points to consider' and can discuss with your doctor the best option, considering the quality of care and reputation of the hospital.

A list of all fertility clinics is available on the Human Fertilization and Embryology Authority (HFEA) website. Currently the choose and book system only allows you to choose the time and place of your first outpatient appointment, though the scheme may be extended. If your fertility clinic is very far away you may be able to have some tests or early treatment at your local hospital.

The amount of money available for the investigation and treatment of subfertility varies across the country, and different areas will have different criteria for eligibility for treatment. For example, there may be restrictions on treatment depending on age, if you have children already, or you may be asked to try a particular medication or treatment.

Everybody has the right to be referred to a specialist for discussion and potential investigation. Your GP will be able to find out the eligibility criteria for treatment in your area. Generally, the NHS aims to pay for one stimulated cycle of in vitro fertilization (IVF) per couple, for women between the ages of 23 and 39. It may be that your particular area may pay for more cycles of a cheaper treatment, such as clomifene ovulation induction or intrauterine insemination (IUI) (see Chapter 7 for more information on treatment options).

Even on the NHS you will be asked to pay prescription charges. At the time of writing, this amounts to £6.85 per medication, so if you are prescribed three medicines on one outpatient prescription, you will be charged £20.55. The true cost of the medication is often significantly more than the £6.85 you are charged, and the NHS covers the difference. You may be exempt from paying these charges if you have certain conditions such as diabetes or a thyroid disorder, or if you are eligible for certain benefits.

It is important to note that waiting lists in the NHS may be long. Once you are seen by your specialist you may have to wait for investigations, wait to be seen by the doctor again, etc. and only then may you be put on the waiting list for treatment.

Remember that fertility treatment does not have to mean IVF. There are many medical, surgical and assisted reproduction treatments, and each area has different criteria as to what you are eligible for. While everyone can ask to be referred to a gynaecologist with respect to subfertility, what is available in terms of investigation and treatment may differ.

If you have been refused treatment or have had up to the limit of treatment available on the NHS, there are schemes that may enable you to afford treatment in the private sector. The 'shared egg scheme' is offered by many clinics. You undergo superovulation, and half of any eggs collected are kept by you and fertilized with your partner's/donor sperm; the other half are given to another woman for fertilization by her partner's/donor sperm. If any of your half of the eggs fertilize and develop they will be transferred back to you; if any of the other half of the eggs develops they will be inserted into the other woman. The couple receiving your eggs will pay the full cost of treatment for both her own and your treatment cycle. You will have no rights to the half of the eggs that you give away; legally you will be treated as an egg donor (see Chapter 9 for more information on donors). In other schemes, donating eggs results in reduced costs.

Private treatment

The cost of private investigations and treatment depends on what you have and where you have it, though costs tend to be similar between clinics. Currently the average cost for one cycle of stimulated IVF is about £4,500. When considering cost, it is important to investigate what is included in the quoted price – does it include consultation fees, investigations, HFEA fees, medications, counselling? If the cost of medications or surgical investigations are excluded, the true cost may be much higher than that quoted. Different procedures cost different amounts; for example, IUI is cheaper than IVF and natural cycles are cheaper than stimulated cycles.

Private health insurers tend not to cover treatment for subfertility. However, they may cover the cost of some of the initial appointments and investigations and in some cases surgery.

Even if you do pay for treatment, you may still be eligible for some treatment on the NHS, for example initial investigations such as blood tests and ultrasound.

Other points to consider

Cost is not the only concern when choosing a clinic. Other issues to consider are:

- Is the clinic licensed by the HFEA? If so, you know it provides legal and safe treatment.
- Where is the clinic? How will you get there? Travel/parking costs?
- Are you eligible for treatment? Some clinics may have age limitations.
- When is payment due?
- What are the opening hours? Does it have evening or Saturday morning opening hours to enable less time away from work?
- What treatments are offered? Do they offer the treatment that is best for you?
- What is the experience of the staff? Does the clinic have experience in treating your specific problem, your specific treatment, your age group?
- How many treatment cycles are cancelled and at what stage?
- What is the multiple birth rate?
- Is embryo freezing and storage offered? If not, how are excess embryos treated?
- What support services are offered? Counselling, support groups? Are they included in the price?
- Would you prefer a small clinic where you may get to know everybody, or a larger clinic that may offer more treatments, etc.?
- Can you see the same doctor each time?
- Go and visit any clinics you are considering, speak to the staff and ask as many questions as you like. The location, ambience, environment, attitude and friendliness of the staff may all influence your decision.

You should consider *success rates* – what are the live birth success rates for a clinic and, specifically, what are the success rates for your age group? Bear in mind, however, that success rates are dependent on many variables; for example a small sample size gives more inaccurate figures than a large sample size. Average success rates are not useful, you need to look at the variables that are specific to you – age, type of causative problem, type of treatment, including whether fresh, frozen or donor eggs/sperm/embryos are used. Look at the type of patients the clinic treats; complicated patients have lower success rates that may bring down average results, but other clinics may only take on simple cases. Check too that what you consider to be success is what is being measured – are they using rates of fertilization, pregnancies or live births?

Affording treatment

There are various methods to decrease the cost of your treatment:

- There may be a discount if you pay as a lump sum instead of spreading the cost of payments. Also, interest may be added if the cost of treatment is spread over a period of time.
- Have some of your initial investigations on the NHS if appropriate. You will need to ask for written documentation of the results.
- Go directly to the drug companies or pharmacies and see if you can obtain the medications you need at a cheaper price than that being offered by the clinic.
- Egg sharing scheme – as described above.

Treatment abroad

You could also have treatment in a clinic outside the UK. These clinics will not be regulated by the HFEA (see below) and may or may not be governed by a regulating body. They may have different procedures regarding numbers of embryos transferred and the screening of donor gametes, and the donor may have different rights to any potential child according to the laws of that country. Therefore it is important to carry out your research into not just the clinic but the laws of the country before starting any treatment abroad.

Fertility and the law

In 1990 the Human Fertilization and Embryology Act was passed by Parliament and the House of Lords. It resulted in the establishment of the Human Fertilization and Embryology Authority (HFEA) to regulate the creation and use of embryos and donated eggs, sperm and embryos. It has various roles including the inspection and publication of reports about clinics and the regulation of research.

Any treatment that involves the act of creating an embryo outside the body is regulated by the HFEA – in vitro fertilization (IVF), intracytoplasmic sperm insertion (ICSI), pre-implantation genetic diagnosis (PGD), zygote intrafallopian transfer (ZIFT) and assisted hatching. Other treatments regulated include the use of donors and surrogates. Treatments where fertilization occurs within the body, for example any artificial insemination such as intrauterine insemination (IUI) or gamete intrafallopian transfer (GIFT), do not have to be regulated. A clinic that is licensed by the HFEA has been inspected and the expertise of its staff and the quality of service and facilities considered appropriate.

Under current UK law, all treatment cycles and resulting live births are registered. When a child born from donated sperm or eggs reaches 18, he or she can ask about the donors. The law also states that clinics must offer counselling and information to patients before receiving treatment, especially if you are donating or receiving sperm, eggs or embryos.

In May 2007, the Human Tissue and Embryos Bill was drafted. It aims to update the Human Fertilization and Embryology Act to reflect the significant changes in medical technology since 1990. One of the aims of the Bill is to replace the HFEA with the Regulatory Authority for Tissue and Embryos (RATE). A further aim is to change the laws regarding the storage of embryos (discussed in Chapter 8, Assisted conception techniques and ethical issues). At the time of writing, the Bill is not law, but is being examined by a parliamentary expert committee. It will then be discussed by both Parliament and the House of Lords, and amendments may be made before it is passed into statute and becomes law.

Welfare of the child assessment

Under the Human Fertilization and Embryology Act of 1990, every person starting treatments where fertilization occurs outside the body must undergo a 'welfare of the child assessment'. This includes IVF, ICSI, PGD, ZIFT and assisted hatching, but not any form of artificial insemination. In some clinics you may undergo the assessment irrespective of the treatment you are receiving. The law states that the welfare of the potential child is paramount.

A common misconception is that the assessment is an attack on your ability or suitability to be a parent. It is not – it aims to make sure that any future child will be safe from physical or psychological harm. However, the assessment is controversial, as it is not carried out in those conceiving naturally. One view is that those having subfertility treatment should not be treated differently from those conceiving naturally; the opposing viewpoint is that the doctors involved in fertility treatment have a responsibility to any children produced.

The assessment can be carried out verbally or on a form. The questions aim broadly to check whether there are any serious problems that may put the child at risk. Topics discussed will include you and your families' medical and psychiatric histories; your ages and ability to look after a child; drug or alcohol abuse; problems with violence; previous involvement with social services and your commitment to bringing up a child. If you are using donated sperm/eggs, they may discuss what you will tell other family members, and the child about his/her origins. The effects of a further child on any existing children will also be considered. The issues discussed will vary depending on your situation, for example, heterosexual, same sex couples, single parents, using your own or donated gametes. Your doctor may ask your permission to obtain further information from your GP or from social services.

If you have already had an assessment for previous fertility treatment you will be reassessed only in certain situations, for example if you have a new partner, or if more than two years have elapsed since your last treatment, in case your situation has changed significantly.

The final decision lies with the 'lead doctor' of the clinic, who is accountable to the Human Fertilization and Embryology Authority. In the majority of cases the assessment will be straightforward and treatment will begin. If treatment is refused, you should be given a full explanation as to why it was refused and any factors that may make the clinic reverse its decision explained. You can make an appeal to the clinic, or if you feel you have been treated unfairly you can make a complaint to the HFEA.

3

How to increase your fertility

Whether you suspect or know you have a problem, are undergoing fertility treatment or simply are just beginning to try to have a baby, there are various steps you can take to increase your chances of becoming pregnant. The aim of this chapter is to give you the knowledge about how to increase your natural fertility, be healthy and help your body to help itself.

> I was in a cycle of appointments, scans, sex on command, medication, more scans, more sex, less sex, no sex, more sex again. I was given loads of advice at the beginning as to what we should be doing and when we should be doing it but as soon as we knew we were 'challenged in the fertility department' I put all that advice aside, and didn't really think it applied any more. Initially, I thought the doctors were going to take care of everything, and that reassured me, but as time went by I began to feel less and less in possession of my own body. Going back and counting my cycle, calculating when I was most fertile, looking after myself, gave me back some control and the feeling that 'I' possessed my body, not the drugs or the doctors, but me. I needed to have command over my own body! (Terri, 28)

Pre-conception

Before you attempt becoming pregnant:

- Start taking folic acid supplements (400mcg/day). Folic acid is a one of the B vitamins. Taking 400mcg of folic acid a day when trying to conceive and until you are 12 weeks pregnant decreases the risk of spina bifida in the baby. These supplements can be bought from most pharmacies and large supermarkets.
- Ask your doctor for a blood test to check whether you are immune to (can't be infected with) rubella, or German measles. You may be immune to rubella if you have been vaccinated or had German measles as a child. If you develop rubella while you are pregnant, it can be dangerous for the developing foetus. If you are not immune, your GP could arrange for you to be vaccinated before you get

pregnant. You should not conceive within three months of the vaccination as it may damage the developing foetus.

- Check if you are due for a smear test. In the UK women are offered smear tests every three years from the age of 25. Treatment of any smear related problems may be more difficult in pregnancy.

When to have sex

If you are able to work out when you ovulate, you are better able to time intercourse when your chances of becoming pregnant are greatest. Any one or a combination of the following methods can be used:

Calculating dates

You can create a menstrual chart to calculate when you ovulate by writing down the date you start your period each month. After a few months you will be able to calculate your cycle length and will know whether or not your cycle is regular. You will ovulate about 14 days before you start your period.

It's obviously easier to work out when you are ovulating if you have a regular cycle. If you have a 28-day cycle you will ovulate around day 14; if you have a 33-day cycle you will ovulate around day 19. From the first day of your period you can then work out when you are next most likely to be ovulating. This method is less likely to work if you have irregular periods.

Basal body temperature

From the time of ovulation to the beginning of menstruation the hormones involved in the menstrual cycle lead to a rise in your temperature. This does not mean that you have a fever or a high temperature. The rise is within the normal range of temperature and you do not necessarily 'feel' hotter. The rise can be detected with an accurate thermometer.

Your temperature may vary very slightly between days. After ovulation there is an increase in temperature of at least 0.2 degrees Celsius (0.4 degrees Fahrenheit) when compared to the first half of the cycle.

You can take your temperature orally, vaginally or rectally but you must take it the same way every day, and at the same time each day. You must take your temperature the moment you wake up, before you do anything else, even go to the toilet or have a drink. As soon as you wake up, take your temperature and record the reading. Unfortunately, there are no lie-ins, as extra sleep can change the reading. Of course you can go back to sleep afterwards!

Start recording your temperature from day 1 of your cycle. It may be easier to plot the readings on a graph so that you can see trends. You can predict that you have ovulated when your temperature is 0.2 degrees Celsius higher than the previous day and stays high for the next three days.

Charting your basal body temperature is a cheap method of calculating ovulation. However, it only tells you when ovulation has occurred, and cannot predict when ovulation will occur. It can also take a few months before patterns emerge.

Cervical mucus examination

Glands inside your cervix produce mucus, the amount and consistency of which changes according to the hormone changes of your menstrual cycle. The mucus becomes thinner around the time of ovulation so that sperm can pass through it on their way to fertilizing an egg. By examining your cervical mucus, it is possible to predict ovulation.

Some women produce more cervical mucus than others and so may be able to assess it by examining their underwear; other women can see it on the toilet paper after wiping and others will have to feel inside their vagina to get a sample. The easiest position to get a sample may be the position in which you insert a tampon, for example, sitting on the toilet or standing with one foot resting on the edge of the toilet or bath. You then insert two clean fingertips into the vagina to obtain a sample. You can check your cervical mucus at any point in the day and can vary the time in the day when the sample is taken.

In the first half of your cycle you may not have very much mucus. This dryness is related to the low hormone levels at the beginning of the cycle. As the level of oestrogen rises, so the amount of mucus you produce will increase, and this is a signal that you are nearing ovulation. Around the time of ovulation the mucus changes, it becomes clear and very stretchy; you can stretch it between your fingers without it breaking. The consistency has been described as being similar to that of raw egg whites. After ovulation as the levels of progesterone rise the mucus changes yet again, becoming cloudy, creamy and much thicker.

- You are in the fertile period of the cycle from when the stretchy mucus appears to about three or four days after the mucus has changed to being thick and sticky.

Charting your cervical mucus is cheap and can be used to predict ovulation, not simply suggest that ovulation has already occurred. However, this test can be unreliable if you are taking certain medications or using lubricants that may affect the mucus. And, as with basal body temperature, charting it may take a few months to be able to recognize the pattern of changes in your mucus, and some women may be uncomfortable with the procedure.

Other signs of your cycle

Some women experience other changes in their bodies that enable them to track their cycles, though they are variable and not always accurate. *Mittelschmerz* literally means 'middle pain' and is the pain felt by some women at ovulation. Other women may recognize mood changes or changes in their breasts which enable them to predict ovulation.

Ovulation prediction kits

Ovulation prediction kits can be bought over the counter from many pharmacies and supermarkets. The most common test, similar to a pregnancy test, involves testing the urine for the LH surge just before ovulation. The test will not tell you if you have ovulated, simply that there is a surge in LH. Ovulation tends to occur about 24–36 hours afterwards. Therefore having sex around this time increases the chance of conception.

The urine test should be taken around the time you expect ovulation to occur and may have to be taken on a few consecutive days before a positive result occurs. If it is taken after ovulation the test will be negative, as it does not test for ovulation, just for the surge of LH. Although easy to use, ovulation prediction kits can be expensive.

Saliva can also be used to test for ovulation, as like cervical mucus it undergoes changes during the monthly cycle. Around ovulation, when examined under a microscope, saliva dries to form patterns that look like ferns. Kits can be obtained that contain a small microscope and slides so you can test your own saliva. Saliva should be tested daily either first thing in the morning, or two hours after brushing your teeth, eating or drinking (as these activities will affect the appearance of the saliva).

How often to have sex

The advice given as to when, and how often, to have sex is designed so that intercourse occurs at the most fertile point of the female cycle (around the time of ovulation) and to maximize the amount of sperm in semen.

Once you have calculated the most fertile time in your cycle, attempt to have sex every other day, for example on days 12, 14, 16 and 18 or days 11, 13, 15 and 17. If you have irregular periods aim for approximately the middle of your cycle.

Having intercourse too often or not often enough can affect the number of sperm in the semen. If a man is ejaculating very regularly the testes cannot maintain sperm production at the rate at which it is being ejaculated, reducing the number of sperm in the semen. Any form of ejaculation, be it from masturbation, oral sex or intercourse, uses up sperm, so on the 'off day' you should not ejaculate. It is also not advisable to 'store' up the sperm, only having intercourse at the time of ovulation, as storing the sperm can result in lower numbers of active, healthy sperm in the semen.

Other factors

Certain lubricants can be harmful to sperm. Do not use a spermicide lubricant while having intercourse. Water-based lubricants such as KY jelly are fine to use but read the label of the lubricant carefully to check it does not contain spermicide.

Certain sexual positions **may** increase the chance of conception. Positions that involve the woman lying down can stop the semen from leaking out of the vagina. The missionary position allows deep penetration and deposits near the cervix increasing the chances of the sperm entering the uterus; alternatively rear-entry (on hands and knees) or side by side positions can be used. Lying with your hips up on a pillow may also help as gravity will enable the semen to pool around the cervix; however, don't lie with your hips up too high as the semen may then collect in the back of the vagina, behind the cervix. Some people advocate lying with your hips on a small pillow for about half an hour after sex to allow the sperm time to enter through the cervix.

Positions that involve the woman straddling the man or standing increase the chance that the semen will run out of the vagina, decreasing the number of sperm available in the right place for conception. It is also important that women do not douche (wash inside the vagina) after intercourse.

Relax. It is well known that putting pressure on a sexual relationship, for example by dictating when, where and how intercourse should be performed, can lead to difficulties within the relationship. It cannot be stressed enough that sex is not just about trying to make a baby, but about the two of you, as a couple, being together. It should be a relaxing, enjoyable experience and not one designed to cause stress. If you can't have sex on day 14, or don't like the missionary position, or have to get up to pee afterwards, it is all right. As long as you are having regular unprotected sex around the time of ovulation you are increasing your chances of conceiving.

Advice for men. To increase your sperm quantity and quality, bear in mind that wearing underpants or clothes that are tight around the groin or taking regular very hot baths can increase the temperature of the testes, resulting in a drop in the sperm count. Regular long training sessions on a bicycle may also affect sperm production.

Home testing kits can assess semen. However, they only measure the concentration of sperm. They check to see if you have over 20 million sperm per millilitre of semen and do not look at the quality of the sperm and therefore do not replace laboratory semen analysis.

Methods to increase your fertility

Aim to be as healthy as you can be in all aspects of your life including diet, exercise and stress levels. These factors affect the fertility of both men and women.

Weight

Your ideal weight will depend on your height. To calculate your Body Mass Index (BMI) divide your weight in kilograms by your height in metres squared (kg/m^2). A healthy BMI is between 20 and 25. Note that muscle is heavier than fat so if you are very muscled you may have a high BMI and still be healthy. If your BMI is under 20 you are underweight, a BMI between 25 and 30 is considered overweight and a BMI over 30 is considered obese. Being both under and overweight has an adverse effect on fertility, as well as on other areas of your health; for example, being overweight is a risk factor for diabetes and heart disease.

Average daily calorie requirements are 2500 kcal for men and 2000 kcal for women. These are average – for example if you are very short you may need fewer calories. Before making major changes to your diet and exercise programme, though, you should consult your doctor.

If you are underweight, weight can be gained without eating unhealthily, for example not eating more junk food but by eating more protein-rich foods or foods rich in 'good' unsaturated fats such as nuts.

If you are overweight, losing weight can be very difficult. The only method that is known to work in the long term involves eating a little less and moving a little more. This means you have to expend more calories than you consume. A healthy, low fat diet combined with exercise should help you lose weight. Start exercise slowly; even little things such as climbing the stairs instead of using the lift, or walking to work instead of taking the bus can make a significant difference. You should aim to lose about 1–2lbs per week. Your GP may be able to refer you to a dietician if you feel it would be helpful.

Even if you are trying to lose weight it is important that you eat breakfast as eating a good breakfast means you are less likely to snack on unhealthy foods later in the morning.

Diet

Even if your BMI is within the normal range you should still eat a healthy diet. A healthy diet is one high in fruit and vegetables and low in fat, especially saturated fat. Beware of food labels that state a food is low in fat, as these foods are often high in sugar and so may still be high in calories. About one third of your diet should be from foods such as cereals, wholegrains and potatoes that release energy slowly.

- Aim to eat at least five portions of fruit and vegetables a day.
- Decrease fat intake by avoiding processed foods such as salamis or pastries. You do need a little fat in your diet but if possible this should be obtained from the good fats, unsaturated fats found in foods such as nuts and avocados.
- Try to avoid eating too much sugar, which is high in calories and may lead to weight gain.
- Aim to drink at least six to eight glasses of liquid a day, about 1.5–2 litres. The best drink is water.
- Aim to eat less salt. Even if you don't add salt to your food, it is found in high levels in processed foods such as breakfast cereals. The current recommendation is that adults do not eat more than 6g of salt per day. Salt is often written as sodium on food labels; multiply the amount of sodium by 2.5 to get the amount of salt in the food.
- Aim for at least two portions of fish a week, one of which should be an oily fish such as salmon. It does not matter if the fish is fresh, frozen, smoked or tinned.
- You may be trying for a baby but at any given time you may not know if you are successful, so you should avoid foods that pregnant women should also avoid. For example, you should not have too many foods rich in vitamin A which can be harmful for your

developing foetus in high levels. Avoid taking vitamin A or fish oil supplements and avoid eating liver or foods made from liver such as liver pâté. Although you should eat fish try to avoid fish high in mercury, which can damage the foetus, such as swordfish, or shark. You should also avoid raw eggs and blue cheeses as they may contain harmful bacteria.

Eating a healthy diet sounds very complicated but actually is not. It does not mean you can never have what you enjoy, be it pizza or chocolate. Everything in moderation – eating healthily is about striking the right balance. This means you can still enjoy having treats, just as long as it isn't every meal time!

Dietary supplements

As mentioned above, all women trying to conceive should be taking supplements of folic acid. Folic acid can be bought alone or in combination with other vitamins and minerals in combination 'pregnancy supplements'.

Pregnant women often become low in iron stores and can become anaemic. You should eat foods rich in iron to build up your body's iron stores before coming pregnant. Foods rich in iron include dark green, leafy vegetables, red meat, pulses and breakfast cereals. Vitamin C helps your body absorb the iron in foods, so try to have a glass of orange juice or other fruit or vegetable when having iron-rich foods.

Some supplements are thought by many people to aid fertility, for example vitamin E with its anti-oxidant properties, or zinc which may help with sperm production. Currently the Department of Health recommends only folic acid as dietary supplementation. It should be possible to get all the other vitamins and minerals needed by eating a healthy diet.

Exercise

Even if your Body Mass Index is within the healthy range it is still important to partake in exercise. This does not have to be hugely strenuous, but should involve getting your heart rate up and burning off some extra calories. Aim for at least 30 minutes of moderate physical activity on most days of the week, and at least three times per week.

Moderate activity is the equivalent of a brisk walk. You should get warm and be slightly out of breath, but still be able to talk to someone without gasping for air. If 30 minutes in one go is too much, split it up into two or three smaller sessions throughout the day. Join a gym or exercise classes at your local borough fitness centre, try a fitness video, walk to work, or do the housework vigorously. You could use it as an opportunity to learn a new skill and meet new people, for example, you and your partner could start dancing lessons.

Keeping fit is an important part of being healthy and therefore fertile. It also has the added benefit that even if you don't feel like it, once you get going, exercise can be relaxing and make you feel really good. It can be used as a way to get rid of stress and so can be especially useful as you start this potentially difficult journey.

Caffeine

Caffeine is found in drinks such as tea, coffee, hot chocolate, cola and chocolate. Currently there is no definitive evidence that caffeine can affect fertility, but the UK Food Standards Agency recommends that pregnant women should have no more than 300mg of caffeine a day, about six cups of tea, or three cups of coffee.

Stopping caffeine altogether can be difficult. Many people are addicted to caffeine without knowing it and get symptoms such as headaches if they miss their morning cup of coffee. Decreasing slowly the amount of caffeine that you consume should help these symptoms. If it is simply the taste that you miss, buy caffeine-free tea, coffee and cola.

Smoking

Many studies have shown that smoking decreases fertility in women. Even passive smoking (breathing in the smoke from other people's cigarettes) can lead to a delay in conceiving. It is well known that smoking while pregnant can affect the developing baby; babies of women who smoke are more likely to be small and have other problems.

Smoking affects not just your fertility, but every aspect of your physical well-being. Among other things, smoking increases your risk of cancers, lung diseases such as emphysema, strokes and heart disease. Smoking is also expensive – at the time of writing, a pack of ten cigarettes cost about £2.50, and a pack of 20 about £5. So, if you smoke ten a day, that is about £17.50 a week, £70 a month and about £900 per year; if you smoke 20 a day the cost doubles to almost £2000 a year – a significant contribution towards fertility treatment!

There is no denying that giving up smoking is hard. Your GP should be able to refer you to a stop smoking programme and support group if you feel it may help. Currently the effect of nicotine replacement patches and other therapies on fertility is not yet known.

Alcohol

The Department of Health recommends that men drink no more than 21 units of alcohol a week and women no more than 14 units. A pint of beer is approximately 2 units, a standard pub measure of spirits one unit, a small glass of wine (125ml) about one and a half units. A bottle of wine (12 per cent) contains about 9 units. You should take into account the size of your wine glasses; the units in 'one glass' are often underestimated, as the glass holds more than you think it does!

The evidence regarding alcohol and subfertility in women is not clear. However, it is well-known that alcohol can damage the developing foetus. The current recommendation is that women who are pregnant or trying to get pregnant should drink no more than one to two units of alcohol per week and should avoid getting drunk to reduce the risk to the baby.

For men, drinking within the recommended limits of 21 units per week has not been shown to affect fertility. However, drinking excessively can affect the quality of semen.

Prescribed drugs

If you are taking prescribed medication, do visit your doctor and explain that you are trying to get pregnant, as various medications, taken by both men and women, can affect fertility, or the developing foetus.

In some cases a difficult decision may have to be made. For example, if you have epilepsy, some anti-convulsants may be known to have a risk of affecting a baby – but badly controlled epilepsy may also affect a developing baby. The decision to stop or change medications should always be made in conjunction with a doctor. Tell your doctor what you are thinking about doing. Even if he or she advises you otherwise, it is important that your doctor is aware of your decision.

Recreational drugs

It is, obviously, advisable to avoid recreational drugs. The effects on fertility are not all known but, for example, cocaine affects the quality of sperm and cannabis can affect your eggs and ovulation.

If you do use recreational drugs, please inform your doctor as he or she may be able to help you to stop. There are various support groups and rehabilitation programmes. You have a right to confidentiality; your doctor is not the same as the police, and no punitive measures will be taken as long as your actions are not putting others at risk.

Being unwell

Fevers and being unwell can adversely affect fertility. Having a high temperature can temporarily lower sperm counts.

Occupation

Some jobs involve exposure to physical and chemical agents that may affect fertility. For example, agricultural workers exposed to the chemicals in pesticides may have affected sperm counts. If you are concerned that your job may be adversely affecting your fertility either visit your GP or, if your company has one, visit your occupational health department for further advice.

Stress

Physical, emotional and mental stress affects us all. Stress can disrupt the female menstrual cycle, even stopping ovulation entirely. The overall effects of stress on fertility are not yet known, but it can be presumed that stress has an adverse effect on fertility as it has an adverse effect on health in general.

Difficult as it can be to relieve stress and tension, talking to each other is important. Talking about your worries and fears not only relieves stress, it also increases your understanding of each other as a couple. If, though, you find that all you talk about are your problems then it may help to talk to a third party, a friend or a counsellor. Taking time out to look after yourselves, to eat well, to have fun, to relax both in and out of each other's company can help ease the stresses involved in both life and trying to have a baby. Try some of the relaxation techniques described later in the book.

Complementary therapy

Herbal medications such as dong quai, or chasteberry (agnus castus) and other complementary therapies such as acupuncture or homeopathy can be used to increase your fertility and to help with any other problems. (See Chapter 11, Complementary treatments and relaxation techniques.)

4

Female causes of subfertility

As you will see from this chapter, causes of subfertility are many and can be complex. They include age, anovulation, ovarian dysfunction and structural problems – problems with the fallopian tubes, fibroids, endometriosis, etc.

Age

One of the reasons why problems with fertility have increased is that the number of women having their first child after the age of 35 has increased dramatically. Women in modern society are faced with tough choices: career or family – it is accepted it is difficult and exhausting to do both full-time. Many women are choosing to focus on another aspect of their lives, or haven't found the right partner. Whatever the reason, many women are waiting to have children.

Girls are born with a finite number of eggs and as you get older there are fewer eggs (the 'ovarian reserve'). Years before the menopause there are age-related changes in the levels of the hormones needed for ovulation. The eggs that are left have aged and may be of a worse quality, have harder shells to prevent penetration by sperm, or have damage to the chromosomes. Simply put, with age, the number of competent, high-quality eggs decreases. Older women are also more likely to have other medical conditions that may affect fertility.

Even ten to 15 years before the average age of menopause (age 50), fertility is reduced. After the age of 40 the chances of conceiving decrease from 20–25 per cent to 5–10 per cent per cycle.

> I am 42 and have never thought of myself as 'old'. I have a busy, exciting life and while I always wanted to have children it was something I thought could wait, that it would happen sometime in the future. Somehow the 'future' has come and I don't have the children I thought I would. Maybe my biological clock was set wrong, but here I am, 42 and now desperate for babies yet being told I'm 'past it'. My advice – start early, don't leave it, it may be too late. And to those who did wait like me, we may be 'old', we may have more complications, we may have lower success rates,

we may have to pay for our treatment, but also, after everything, we may still be able to have our babies. The doctors say the chances are lower than average – but even if they said I had a 1 per cent chance I would do it; in comparison to nothing, which my chances are without help, one per cent is huge, it could mean the world to me. Of course, I want to take my chance! I'm on my second cycle of IVF now, crossing fingers and toes and hoping for the best. (Anne, 42)

Diagnosis

A diagnosis of subfertility related to age and therefore decreasing numbers of eggs is made by:

- Age
- Blood tests – the levels of FSH at the beginning of a cycle become raised. Levels over 10 international units/litre (IU/L) indicate reduced ovarian reserve, levels over 40 IU/L indicate that the ovary is no longer functioning.
- Other areas relating to subfertility should also be investigated and treated as appropriate.

Treatment

- IVF or donor IVF (see Chapters 8 and 9).

Unfortunately success rates even with assisted reproductive techniques are lower in older women and many centres have an upper age limit.

I realize that it all sounds very gloomy. While hoping for the best, however difficult it may be, you should realize that the treatments have a lower chance of working than in younger women. Treatments do work in some cases but it is important to be realistic, while at the same time trying to remain optimistic. Do also have a look back at Chapter 3, How to increase your fertility.

Anovulation

Anovulation is when no egg is released from the ovary during the monthly cycle and is characterized by infrequent periods (oligomenorrhoea) or absent periods (amenorrhoea). A cycle length longer than 35 days or shorter than 21 days is suggestive of anovulation. Fertility problems are due to disorders of ovulation in approximately 30 per cent of couples.

Diagnosis

- Via a blood test for progesterone – levels of progesterone above 30nmol/l indicate that ovulation has taken place. The test should be taken when levels are highest, seven days before your period is due.
- Ultrasound – transvaginal ultrasound is used to follow and measure a follicle in the ovary as it increases in size and then collapses and shrinks after ovulation.
- Over the counter kits and self-evaluation (see Chapter 3, How to increase your fertility).

Causes of anovulation

I have divided the causes below into two sections: the first is a disruption of hormonal control at the level of the brain: hypothalamic-pituitary causes; and the second is about problems at the level of the ovaries.

Hormonal control in the brain – hypothalamic-pituitary causes

The hypothalamus and pituitary gland work together to form the hypothalamic-pituitary axis. The hypothalamus secretes GnRH, stimulating the pituitary to secrete FSH and LH, without which ovulation cannot take place.

Hypogonadotrophic hypogonadism

This means a lack of sex hormones that leads to the ovaries not functioning. It can be caused by hypothalamus or pituitary gland failure. The end result is that LH and FSH are not secreted so ovulation does not occur.

Causes

- Low body weight (Body Mass Index (BMI) below 19 or 20). Reasons for being underweight may include poor diet or malnutrition, excessive exercise or eating disorders such as anorexia nervosa or bulimia nervosa. Some women are simply very slim. Those who are underweight or exercise excessively produce lower levels of gonadotrophin releasing hormone and thus do not ovulate.
- Being overweight (having a BMI between 25 and 30) or obese (obesity is defined as a BMI above 30). Being overweight leads to a decrease in GnRH production and therefore, anovulation.

Treatment

- Adjustments in diet to return body weight to the normal Body Mass Index range of 20–25; this should lead to ovulation.
- Ovulation induction (see Chapter 7, Medical and surgical treatment).

Hyperprolactinaemia

This is excess production of the hormone prolactin (a hormone produced by the pituitary in the production of breast milk). When levels of prolactin become too high, they decrease levels of LH and FSH, so stopping ovulation. Hyperprolactinaemia is generally caused by a benign tumour of the pituitary gland.

Symptoms

- Secondary amenorrhoea – initially having regular periods but these then becoming irregular or stopping.
- You may produce and leak breast milk (galactorrhoea).
- Occasionally you may get headaches or disturbances of vision. If this occurs you must visit your doctor urgently as this can indicate that the overgrowth of the pituitary gland may need removing.

Diagnosis

- Blood test – high levels of prolactin.
- MRI or CT scan – used to detect the overgrowth in the pituitary.

Treatment

- A medication called bromocriptine acts on a receptor in the brain to lower the levels of prolactin. As the prolactin levels fall your periods should return. In 70–80 per cent of women ovulation then occurs.
- Ovulation induction could also be appropriate (see Chapter 7, Medical and surgical treatment).

Chronic disease

Any chronic disease can lead to anovulation by reducing hormone production. Diseases involving other hormones, such as high or low levels of steroid production from the adrenal glands, can result in anovulation. Treating the condition may lead to an improvement in fertility.

Stress

Anovulation can be caused by stress, which can be physical such as chronic disease. Physical stress may lead to weight loss or malnourishment. Emotional stress can also lead to anovulation. Many women report that their periods become infrequent during times of stress.

> I wouldn't have described myself as 'stressed', at least no more stressed than anybody else I know who juggles the demands of relationships, friends, family and work and finding time to go the gym! It was only when I wanted to have a baby that I

really started paying any attention to my periods at all, except as a painful nuisance. They were just always there, unless I had an exam, or a deadline, or went on an aeroplane, or my gran passed on ... and then I realized that whenever things became a bit difficult, my period didn't come, or was late. Quite frankly, I was always so caught up in whatever it was I barely noticed. All my friends agreed, if you were a bit stressed you don't get your period.

So then we wanted to try for a baby. How can you not get stressed about it? It becomes the only thing you think about! Of course, the more I thought, the more irregular I became, so I couldn't even work out which day I was supposed to be ovulating! The wait for a period turned into a mass of conflicting feelings – if I had a period then at least I had ovulated, but then I wasn't pregnant and if the period didn't come did this mean that I wasn't ovulating, or, dare I even think it, could I be pregnant? Round and round we went.

Everyone said if I relaxed it would happen, why didn't I take a holiday? So we went away – but holidays are only relaxing if you can escape whatever it is that is making you stressed, such as work. There is no escape from wanting and waiting for a baby! I have started yoga classes to help me to relax, we are still trying! (Claire, 31)

Treatment

- Ovulation induction.
- Stress related anovulation may also be helped by counselling or cognitive behavioural therapy.

Idiopathic

Idiopathic means that no cause can be found for the condition; in this situation, no reason has been found for your anovulation. Again, ovulation induction can be used.

Rarer causes of anovulation

Sheehan's syndrome (panhypopituitarism) – caused by a lack of blood supply to the pituitary, for example after a large haemorrhage or trauma. None of the hormones of the pituitary are produced, leading to symptoms such as fatigue or loss of pubic hair as well as absent periods.

Kallman's syndrome – here the hypothalamus does not produce GnRH. Symptoms include a reduced sense of smell.

Cerebral irradiation/surgery – removal of the pituitary by surgery or radiation (after a pituitary tumour or treatment for leukaemia). No hormones can be produced, leading to anovulation.

Ovulation induction can be used for these rarer causes.

Thyroid disease

The thyroid gland is in the neck and produces the hormone thyroxine which is involved in many processes in the body. The hypothalamus produces thyrotrophin releasing hormone (TRH), which stimulates the pituitary gland to secrete thyroid stimulating hormone (TSH), which in turn stimulates the thyroid gland to produce thyroxine.

Hypothyroidism Hypothyroidism is when not enough thyroxine is produced. The low levels of thyroxine cause the hypothalamus to secrete high levels of TRH, which also stimulate production of prolactin. The high levels of prolactin decrease levels of FSH and LH and therefore ovulation can-not take place.

Symptoms include

- cold intolerance
- fatigue and lethargy
- dry thin hair and dry skin
- weight gain or difficulty in losing weight
- depression
- decreased libido
- irregular or absent periods.

Diagnosis is by blood tests and treatment is with replacement thyroxine to lower the levels of TRH and therefore prolactin, hopefully restarting the menstrual cycle. Ovulation induction or IVF may be used.

Hyperthyroidism Hyperthyroidism means that too much thyroxine is produced, which can disrupt ovulation by reducing the active levels of sex hormones.

Symptoms include

- heat intolerance
- weight loss despite increased appetite
- restlessness and irritability
- palpitations
- decreased libido.

Again, it is diagnosed by blood tests. Anti-thyroid drugs, radioactive iodine or surgery may be used to treat it, and, again, ovulation induction or IVF may be suitable fertility treatments.

Ovarian dysfunction

This is when, even though the hormones of the brain are being produced, the ovaries cannot respond to produce an egg. There may be a number of reasons for this.

Polycystic ovarian syndrome

Polycystic ovarian syndrome (PCOS) is the most common cause of failure of ovulation, affecting 70 per cent of women with subfertility due to anovulation. Women with polycystic ovarian syndrome have many cysts (small fluid-filled sacs) in their ovaries, and changes in their hormone levels. The cysts alone occur in up to 20 per cent of women and are termed polycystic ovaries (PCO), not PCOS. Women with simple polycystic ovaries will have no symptoms and should not have problems ovulating.

The hormone changes in PCOS are complicated. High levels of testosterone result in many small follicles being stimulated each month but one dominant follicle does not form and therefore ovulation does not occur. There is also a link between insulin (the hormone involved in controlling the levels of sugar in the blood) and PCOS. These changes mean that women with PCOS are more likely to be overweight and find it difficult to lose weight.

> As a teenager I was always a bit overweight, had irregular periods and bad skin – who didn't? I assumed I would grow out of it. It was only when I began to notice dark hairs appearing where they shouldn't that I went to the doctor, which was when they discovered I had PCOS. It was good to know why it seemed hard for me to lose weight. I researched PCOS until I could have written a book myself and devoured gossip magazines where they tell you that celebrity X has PCOS and managed to have children.
>
> I didn't wait – after four months of trying to get pregnant I went to my doctor saying that as I had PCOS I wanted to be referred to a fertility doctor, and he obliged. I was shocked to discover that my BMI was 36, and I was technically obese. After all the investigations were done the answer according to the experts was simple – the treatments won't work unless you lose weight. Easier said than done. They referred me to a dietician and got me

cheaper membership at a gym and little by little the weight came off, and as they said, my periods began to become more regular. I still needed clomifene to ovulate and now have two children. My BMI is now 27, I try my best to keep my weight down as I know I have a higher chance of having diabetes and other problems, but it is hard. It was easy to blame any weight gain on the PCOS but I eventually realized I was going to have to put in the work to help the doctors help me. (Mary, 36)

Symptoms

- Overweight (and difficulties losing weight)
- Spotty skin (acne)
- Unwanted hair on the face or body
- Irregular or absent periods

Diagnosis

Ultrasound – cysts are seen as a 'necklace of beads' around the ovary. The 'beads' will be black (fluid), with a rim of white (the sac). Blood tests can check hormone levels, for example, the balance of FSH and LH may change and high levels of testosterone and prolactin may be found.

Treatment

- Weight loss (see Chapter 3, How to increase your fertility) – a drop in body weight can change the levels of hormones and in some cases may be all that is needed to kickstart ovulation.
- Metformin is a medication originally used for treating diabetes. It works to help the body to use up sugar and may make you less hungry. Metformin helps people to lose weight and helps women with PCOS who are not overweight, though how it does this is not yet known. Side effects include nausea, vomiting, diarrhoea and tummy pain. These often disappear with time.
- PCOS anovulation can be treated with ovulation induction, IUI or IVF (see Chapters 7 and 8).

Premature ovarian failure (premature menopause)

The menopause is the last period, after which the ovaries no longer produce eggs. Preceding the menopause, ovulation and therefore menstruation become infrequent. The average age of menopause in the western world is 50.

Premature menopause occurs when the last period has taken place before the age of 40 or 45. Your ovaries have stopped producing eggs earlier than they should. This affects one in 10,000 women under 20, 1 per cent of women under 40 and up to 15 per cent of the female population under the age of 45.

Causes of premature menopause may include autoimmune disorders, such as rheumatoid arthritis and systemic lupus erythematosus, where the body's immune system mistakenly begins to attack itself. In this case the body attacks the ovaries.

Premature menopause will occur if you have undergone surgery to remove *both* of your ovaries due to certain cysts or ovarian cancer. Chemotherapy and radiotherapy can also affect the ovaries. Chemotherapy affects the entire body so even if the cancer is not in the pelvis, the drugs used may damage the ovaries. Radiotherapy uses radiation to destroy cancer. It is directed at the relevant area of the body, so if the cancer is in the pelvis the ovaries may receive radiation and be damaged. Rarely infections such as mumps can cause premature ovarian failure.

Finally, some cases are idiopathic (i.e. we don't know why they have occurred). A cause cannot be found in many women with the premature menopause. Theories include an unknown viral infection, genetic causes or environmental toxins.

Symptoms

Apart from irregular or absent periods, symptoms are related to decreased oestrogen levels and include

- hot flushes
- mood swings
- irritability and mood changes including depression
- decreased libido
- vaginal dryness (which may lead to irritation or painful sexual intercourse)
- weight gain
- insomnia or disrupted sleep
- dry skin and thinning hair.

> I was 26 when my periods became irregular, and when I turned 29 they stopped entirely. My GP took blood tests and told me I had the results of a woman in her 50s. The gynaecologist told me I had entered the menopause early. That was it, 29 and game over. I hadn't even thought about having children, I didn't even have a long-term partner and yet I was being told it would never happen for me and they didn't know why. Suddenly having a baby was the only thing I could think about and I had never really thought

about it before except by trying not to get pregnant. The only way I can ever get pregnant is by donor egg IVF and donor eggs are hard to find. The other aspects such as the increased risk of osteoporosis, I barely even considered. Four years on I have found a partner. Telling him was awful, I felt I had to tell him at a stage in our relationship where we weren't even serious as I didn't want him to feel that he had been 'tricked' into a relationship with someone who knew they couldn't give him something he may have wanted. Thankfully he said all he wanted was me, but I still don't know if just the two of us is enough for me. We are looking into adoption and fostering. (Nita, 33)

Diagnosis

Blood tests can pick up low progesterone levels in the second half of your cycle, while levels of follicle stimulating hormone and luteinizing hormones will be high.

Treatment

- IVF, generally donor egg IVF.
- If you are going to have your ovaries removed, or have chemotherapy or radiotherapy, it may be possible to retrieve and freeze some of your eggs beforehand to use in IVF.
- Hormone replacement therapy (HRT) may help prevent osteoporosis and relieve menopausal symptoms. Herbal remedies include agnus castus (chasteberry) or black cohosh.

Genetic (inherited) causes of ovarian dysfunction

Genetic diseases may be identified by looking at the structure of the DNA in your cells (karotyping). These syndromes include Turner's syndrome in which the ovaries are underdeveloped and cannot produce eggs and androgen insensitivity syndrome (AIS or testicular feminization) in which there are no ovaries.

Problems with the fallopian tubes

The egg becomes fertilized by sperm within the fallopian tube on its way to the uterus. The tubes have many other functions. They have a role in the maturation of sperm and in nourishing the fertilized egg. In order to do this, they need to be both unblocked (patent) and functioning. Problems with the tubes occur in up to one third of couples with fertility problems.

Infection is the most common cause of tubal damage. The extent of the damage depends on the severity of the infection and the number of times the tubes have been affected. Infection may lead to the formation of adhesions, bits of scar tissue that block the tubes. Tubes can become infected due to sexually transmitted diseases (STDs) such as chlamydia and gonorrhoea, post-pregnancy infection or after pelvic surgery such as an abortion or hysteroscopy.

> Everyone says it isn't your fault that you are infertile. But what if it really is your fault – it is absolutely mine! I had a boyfriend who gave me chlamydia. It was treated but years on I haven't got pregnant and the doctors say my tubes are blocked. It has taken a lot of therapy for the feelings of guilt to begin to go away – I still feel the situation my partner and I are in is my fault – if only I hadn't met my ex, if only I hadn't trusted him, if only we had used condoms, if only I got tested earlier, if only, if only! I am on the waiting list for surgery to try to unblock the tubes. (Charmaine, 33)

The tubes may also become blocked after an ectopic pregnancy, any pelvic surgery, including female sterilization, or due to endometriosis.

Tubal damage from infection can be prevented by practising safe sex using condoms, having regular screening for STDs and treating any infection with antibiotics. If you have been infected, encourage your partner to get tested and treated otherwise he may simply pass the infection back to you.

Having problems with your tubes will not cause any symptoms apart from problems in getting pregnant.

Diagnosis

- Screening for STDs
- Hysterosalpingography
- Hysterosalpingo-contrast sonography
- Laparoscopy and dye examination

(For more information, see Chapter 6, Diagnostic tests.)

Treatment

- Surgery – reversal of sterilization, adhesiolysis (breaking down the adhesions), tubal recannulation
- IVF
- If there is irreversible tubal damage it is recommended that the tube/s are removed in order to increase the chances of successful IVF.

(See Chapter 7, Medical and surgical treatment.)

Other problems within the pelvis

Fibroids

Fibroids are very common benign overgrowths of the muscle of the uterus, that can bulge into the cavity of the uterus. Why fibroids may result in fertility problems is not yet known, but the most likely reason is they reduce the chances of implantation; rarely, a fibroid may block the tubes. It is estimated that fibroids are involved in subfertility in up to 10 per cent of women; they also carry an increased risk of miscarriage.

Symptoms may include a feeling of 'fullness' or a lump in the abdomen, heavy periods, bleeding between periods, passing urine very frequently or incontinence, due to pressure on the bladder by the fibroid/s. Occasionally fibroids can degenerate or twist, causing acute pain.

Diagnosis

- 'Bulkiness' on vaginal examination
- Ultrasound scan
- Hysteroscopy
- Laparoscopy

(See Chapter 6, Diagnostic tests.)

Treatment

- Stopping ovulation with medication shrinks fibroids but obviously cannot be used if you are trying to get pregnant! The fibroids may grow again once the medications are stopped.
- Myomectomy – surgery to remove fibroids from the womb. If fibroids are the only contributing factor to subfertility, chances of spontaneous pregnancy afterwards are approximately 60 per cent.
- Fibroid embolization – a clot is sent into the artery supplying the fibroid, cutting off its blood supply.
- IVF – fibroids are associated with a lower live birth rate in IVF. This may be due to difficulties in implantation or due to miscarriage.

Endometriosis

This is when cells similar to those in the lining of the womb are present outside the uterus, for example, behind the ovaries. These cells respond to the hormones of the menstrual cycle and are shed each month causing pain, typically just before a period, and can form cysts. With time the shedding causes adhesions in the pelvis, which can lead to blockage of the tubes and result in subfertility.

Between one and two fifths of women with subfertility may have endometriosis but this may not be the most significant contributing factor. Five per cent of fertile women have endometriosis.

Symptoms may include pain before or during periods, abdominal pain during or after sex, and chronic pelvic pain.

Diagnosis

- Tenderness or bulkiness on vaginal examination
- Ultrasound scan – may show cysts
- Laparoscopy

(See Chapter 6, Diagnostic tests.)

Treatment

Medications for endometriosis suppress ovulation and therefore cannot be used.

- Endometriosis without damage to the tubes – ovulation induction and/or IUI
- Mild endometriosis – surgery to remove the endometriosis by excision or laser
- Severe endometriosis – IVF
- Surgery to break down adhesions

(For more information see Chapter 7, Medical and surgical treatment).

Cervical problems

The cervix is the neck of the womb and is at the top of the vagina. It has a tiny canal through which sperm have to swim to enter the womb.

There may be problems with cervical mucus. The cervix produces mucus which becomes watery around ovulation to allow sperm to enter the womb. In cervical mucus hostility the sperm cannot penetrate the mucus. It can occur if there is not enough oestrogen stimulation to the cervix or if the cervix has been damaged due to scarring or infection.

The cervical mucus may contain anti-sperm antibodies which may result in the sperm being destroyed. These can be tested for using a blood test. The theory of anti-sperm antibodies in subfertility is, as yet, unproven. Cervical mucus hostility is a controversial issue among subfertility doctors.

Rarely, the cervical canal can be narrowed (stenotic) or scarred and blocked, for example after surgery to the cervix such as laser treatments for abnormal smear tests.

Diagnosis

Post-coital test – not recommended routinely (see Chapter 6, Diagnostic tests).

Treatment

- Intra-uterine insemination (IUI)
- IVF
- GIFT/ZIFT

(See Chapter 8, Assisted conception techniques and ethical issues.)

Recurrent miscarriage

Miscarriage is very common, ending 15–25 per cent of pregnancies, most before 12 weeks of pregnancy. Recurrent miscarriage is defined as having at least three miscarriages in succession with the same partner. The problem is not with conception but with staying pregnant; however, the end result is the same as for any of the causes of subfertility – no baby. If you are experiencing recurrent miscarriage you may experience any of the emotions talked about in this book. Whether or not you were able to get pregnant must feel to you almost irrelevant – you don't have the baby that you desire. The medical profession considers recurrent miscarriage separate to fertility problems as it has different causes and treatments. Despite this I hope that you will find sections of this book useful.

Recurrent miscarriage occurs in one in 100 couples. In the next pregnancy the chance of miscarriage is still low, approximately 4 in 10, but after three miscarriages it may be helpful to undergo investigation.

Possible causes

Auto-immune disease is thought in some cases to cause blood clots in the placenta, which prevent it working. Diagnosis is by blood tests, and treatment with aspirin or injections to keep the blood thin and prevent the clots forming.

Anatomical reasons Conditions which result in distortion of the cavity of the uterus and prevent it growing with the foetus such as fibroids can cause recurrent miscarriage.

Cervical incompetence is when the cervix is weak and opens too early. It tends to cause late miscarriage. A stitch can sometimes be put in to strengthen the cervix after 12 weeks of pregnancy.

Polycystic ovarian syndrome How this causes miscarriage is not known but the risks of miscarriage may be decreased with the diabetes medication metformin.

Clotting disorders can increase the likelihood of blood clots in the placenta.

Chromosomal defects Humans have 46 chromosomes within each of their cells, which carry their genes: 23 chromosomes come from the mother and 23 from the father. An imbalance or incorrect number of chromosomes in a foetus increases the chances of miscarriage. Some people may carry a chromosomal imbalance which does not affect them, but may cause an imbalance in a foetus that results in miscarriage. You can be tested for this with a blood test; treatment offered may include pre-implantation genetic diagnosis.

Smoking and *obesity* have also been linked to recurrent miscarriage.

For more information on diagnosis and treatment of recurrent miscarriage please see your GP.

5

Male causes of subfertility

Male factors are involved in approximately half of subfertile couples, though they may not be the only factor. Problems with fertility affect 20 per cent of men. This may come as a surprise to some men.

> I had always assumed it was her problem. Not her problem in that I wasn't affected, but in that there was nothing wrong with me! When they said they had to test my sperm I was actively surprised. Why would they want to test my sperm, it's fine, I thought, I've been producing it for years, I've got great swimmers. I felt they were questioning my very manhood by questioning my little men. I was man, low of voice, hairy of chest, hunter, provider – of course my sperm were up for it! I was so sure of myself that I only produced the sample to prove them wrong. Only I was wrong and there weren't as many swimmers as there should have been and now we have to try IUI. (Keiran, 37)

The cornerstone of the investigation of male subfertility is the examination of the sperm (semen analysis).

Semen analysis

The sperm and the semen are examined. Ideally samples are produced by masturbation, after three days of abstinence from ejaculation. At the clinic you will be given an appropriate pot (you are not expected to fill it up, the average man produces approximately 2–5ml of semen with each ejaculation). You should not use lubricant. You may produce your sample at home if you can bring it into the laboratory within an hour of being produced. If you have a religious objection to or difficulty with masturbation please discuss this with your doctor. In these circumstances the sample may be provided after sexual intercourse using a non-spermicidal condom.

> It was so embarrassing, I felt everyone in the waiting room knew that I was going to have to go and produce a sample. It is just not something you normally do in a hospital. I worried I would be so

> anxious about it and the results of the test that I wouldn't be able to perform. (Sam, 33)

Unless your sample is completely normal you will be asked to repeat the test after a six-week gap as there are many reasons for a transient drop in sperm counts. Sperm are analysed for both quantity and quality.

Causes of male subfertility

Causes of male subfertility are wide-ranging and include problems with both sperm production and transport of sperm.

Problems with sperm production

Sperm production is controlled by hormone production in the brain (hypothalamic-pituitary axis) and in the testes. Irrespective of the cause of the hormonal problem, the symptoms will be those of low levels of testosterone, which vary according to when the low levels of testosterone first started: if the deficiency is lifelong or starts at puberty the testicles will be underdeveloped and there will be a lack of body hair. If it starts in adulthood, body hair and muscle strength will be lost, there may be depression, mood swings, decreased libido and impotence.

Low levels of testosterone result in decreased production of sperm; in some cases no sperm may be produced. Disorders of sperm number are often associated with disorders of sperm quality.

Diagnosis

- Blood tests – low levels of FSH and testosterone indicate a hypothalamic or pituitary problem.
- Normal or high levels of FSH with low testosterone levels indicate a problem within the testes.
- Testicular biopsy – to see if any sperm are being made. Sperm may be produced but in too few numbers to be seen on semen analysis.

Hormonal causes in the brain of problems of sperm production

Hypogonadotrophic hypogonadism

This is a rare condition in which the testes are functioning normally but they are not being stimulated by the hormones of the hypothalamus or pituitary. Without stimulation of GnRH, or FSH and LH, testosterone is not produced and therefore sperm production is decreased. This is treated with hormone replacement with gonadotrophins (sex hormones).

Hyperprolactinaemia

High levels of prolactin lead to a decrease in the levels of LH and FSH produced and thus a decrease in sperm production. It is generally caused by a benign tumour of the pituitary gland.

Symptoms include impotence and changes in libido; decreased or absent sperm in semen; development of breasts and production of breast milk. If you get headaches or disturbances of vision, visit your doctor urgently as the overgrowth may need to be removed. Hyperprolactinaemia is diagnosed with blood tests showing high levels of prolactin. MRI or CT scans are used to detect the overgrowth in the pituitary.

Treatment involves the medication bromocriptine to lower the levels of prolactin, or surgery may be undertaken to remove the tumour.

Hypothyroidism

Low levels of thyroid hormone result in high levels of prolactin being produced, decreasing the amount of FSH and LH and thus causing problems with the production of sperm. Symptoms include decreased/ absent sperm production; decreased libido; cold intolerance; fatigue and lethargy; weight gain or difficulty in losing weight; and depression.

Hypothyroidism is diagnosed with a blood test which shows low levels of thyroid hormone and high levels of TSH. It is treated with thyroxine replacement.

Causes of problems with sperm production in the testes

Sometimes, FSH and LH are being produced as normal but the testes cannot produce sperm. This may happen for a number of reasons:

Cryptorchidism The testes have not descended into the scrotum and may not function properly even if surgery has been undertaken to bring the testes back into the scrotum.

Genetic causes Up to 7 per cent of subfertile men have a genetic cause such as Klinefelter's syndrome (47 XXY), when every cell has an extra X chromosome. The men tend to be tall and thin with small testes.

Chemotherapy drugs or radiotherapy These can damage the testes. Sperm can be frozen (cryopreservation) prior to treatment for future use in IVF or ICSI. See relevant chapters.

Trauma Even minor injuries such as sport injuries can lead to swelling of, or bleeding in, the testicles. If severe, permanent damage to sperm production may result.

Torsion The testis twists cutting off its own blood supply resulting in damage unless treated quickly by surgery.

Infection Orchitis, inflammation of the testes, can result in testicular damage causing a failure of sperm production. It can be caused by infections such as mumps if it affects the testicles.

Too frequent ejaculation Ejaculation at least once every day may mean that sperm cannot be produced quickly enough to keep up with how fast it is being used up, decreasing the amount of sperm in the semen.

Heat The testicles are in the scrotum, as sperm production requires a lower temperature than that of the body. Wearing tight underwear or having regular very hot baths can increase the temperature of the testicles and affect both sperm numbers and quality.

Idiopathic Most cases of mild to moderate decrease in sperm numbers do not have an obvious cause. Some may be related to fevers or major illnesses that can cause a temporary drop in sperm production. It may improve without treatment.

Age While the effect of age on women's fertility is well known, there is much less evidence about the effect of age on men's fertility, and many men father children in later life. However, increasing age could result in lower levels of hormones, decreased functioning of the testicles and therefore decreased sperm production.

Treatment Treatment depends on the number and quality of any sperm produced and includes IUI, IVF and ICSI; donor sperm may be used.

Varicocele

A varicocele is a dilation of the veins within the testicles that may lead to a decrease in sperm production. Symptoms may include a feeling of heaviness in the testicle.

Varicoceles are controversial among fertility experts as they occur in both fertile and infertile men. It may be that the varicocele is only one part of the problem. If the varicocele has been present during childhood and puberty the testis may not have developed properly. Alternatively the increased temperature caused by the abnormal blood flow in the testicle or pressure on the testicle may decrease sperm production.

Varicoceles are diagnosed by examination of the testicles and ultrasound scan.

Treatment

- Surgery – the varicocele is tied off or removed.
- Embolization – a clot is sent down the veins of the varicocele, cutting off its oxygen and nutrient supply.

Surgery should result in the improvement of sperm quality, but there is not much evidence to suggest that it increases pregnancy rates. Alternatively, as above, IUI, IVF, ICSI or donor sperm can be used.

Problems with the transport of sperm

The tubes that carry the sperm from the testicles to the penis (epididymis and vas deferens) may be blocked or absent.

Again, there are several possible causes:

- previous surgery to the groin or abdomen, including hernia operations and operations to bring down undescended testicles;
- trauma, even minor trauma like minor sporting injuries;
- hernias extending into the scrotum;
- previous vasectomy/sterilization;
- absence of the vas deferens – this is more common in men who have cystic fibrosis. It is treated with sperm retrieval techniques for use in ICSI;
- infections – sexually transmitted diseases such as chlamydia and gonorrhoea can cause obstruction. These can be asymptomatic or present with discharge. Swabs are taken to diagnose the infection and antibiotics given.

Diagnosis

- Blood tests – normal levels of FSH and testosterone
- Scrotal or transrectal ultrasound
- Vasography

For more information, please see Chapter 6, Diagnostic tests.

Treatment

- Surgery to reverse a vasectomy or bypass an obstruction. Sperm are being produced so once the obstruction is removed sperm should appear in the ejaculate.
- Sperm can be retrieved from the testes with surgical techniques for use in ICSI or IVF.
- Donor sperm can be used.

For more information on any of the above treatment options, see Chapter 7, Medical and surgical treatment.

Immunological causes

The immune system is the body's defence system, but occasionally it can act against cells of the body. In fertility problems, the immune system may act against sperm by producing anti-sperm antibodies. The antibodies may destroy or damage sperm, though this topic is currently controversial due to a lack of evidence to support these theories.

It is diagnosed by semen analysis – immunobead testing to detect antibodies.

Treatment

- Medication – steroids can dampen down the immune system and stop the production of anti-sperm antibodies.
- Sperm obtained through masturbation can be 'washed', removing any antibodies, and then used in assisted reproductive techniques.

For more information please see Chapter 7, Medical and surgical treatment.

Problems with sexual function

Impotence is when a man cannot have sexual intercourse, due to either failure of erection or failure of ejaculation. Sperm production is generally normal, but the sperm are not placed within the woman. Occasional problems with erections are very common, though, and do not mean that there is a long-term problem.

Erectile dysfunction (ED)

Erectile dysfunction is an inability to have an erection for long enough to have intercourse and ejaculation. It can be caused by physiological or psychological problems or a combination, as anxiety can then exacerbate a physiological problem.

> I am well aware of my shortcomings in the bedroom, but when it began to affect not only our sex life but our ability to have children, I knew we had to take action. Months of sex counselling later we are managing, now we are crossing our fingers and waiting to fall pregnant. (Dave, 36)

Physiological causes

During arousal the brain sends signals to the penis via nerves to dilate the blood vessels and allow the penis to fill with blood and become erect.

- Problems with the blood supply – the blood vessels that supply the penis can become narrow and hardened, preventing blood from entering the penis. Alternatively, the vessels may not be able to keep the blood in the penis, resulting in an inability to sustain an erection.
- Problems with the nerves – an injury to the nervous system such as a stroke, spinal cord injury or multiple sclerosis.
- Trauma to the pelvis – for example after an injury or surgery, or radiotherapy.
- Hormone problems – testosterone deficiency can lead to a loss of sexual desire and libido and ED.
- Drugs – many drugs such as high blood pressure medication, anti-depressants and alcohol can have adverse effects.

Psychological causes

Depression, anxiety and stress can all result in erectile dysfunction. Other causes include confusion regarding sexual orientation, conflict with partner, sexual boredom and previous problems in a sexual relationship. A cycle may be entered in which an inability to produce an erection on one occasion results in worry that it will happen again, worsening the problem.

Treatment

- Counselling or sex therapy to treat any psychological component. This can be useful even if you feel the problem is physiological as stress may worsen the situation.
- Medication – the most famous example is Viagra (sildenafil). Viagra works by increasing the blood flow to the penis. Some of the drugs may result in poor sperm quality.
- Surgery – may involve rewiring the blood supply to the penis to avoid any blockages, or the insertion of implants. Sperm can be harvested from the testicles for use in assisted reproductive techniques.
- Occasionally semen can be obtained with a vibrator or rectal stimulation in men who have problems with the nerves supplying the penis, such as in spinal cord injuries, for use in assisted reproductive techniques.

Premature ejaculation

Premature ejaculation means ejaculating earlier than you and/or your partner would like. It is very common and probably affects the majority of men on at least one occasion. It is only a concern in subfertility if it prevents vaginal penetration.

Counselling may help relieve the pressure on the man to perform, and lessen stress, which probably worsens the condition. Advice can be given regarding various exercises to delay ejaculation. Any collected sperm can be used in IUI or IVF.

Retrograde ejaculation

Retrograde ejaculation is when the semen does not come out through the penis but instead is released backwards into the bladder. A sphincter at the neck of the bladder is designed to prevent retrograde ejaculation. However, it may be damaged after surgery, or in conditions such as diabetes.

The sperm can be retrieved from the urine and then used in IUI (see Chapter 8, Assisted conception techniques and ethical issues). The acidity of the urine may damage sperm and so is neutralized with oral medication (sodium bicarbonate).

6

Diagnostic tests

When you and your partner visit your doctor you will be able to see which, if any, of the following tests are needed. A common misconception is that once you are in the hospital system, treatment can be started straightaway. This is not appropriate as investigations are needed to guide doctors to the cause of the problem and therefore to the best treatment. Sometimes, too, the results of one test lead doctors to ask for a further test. Not all centres offer all the investigations described below.

> I was so frustrated I could have screamed. I had already waited six weeks to see a gynaecologist and then had to wait at least a month to get all the blood tests done at the right part of my cycle. My ultrasound was done during that first month but then I had to wait for six weeks for my husband's second sperm sample, and then to be put on the waiting list for a special kind of x-ray of my womb and tubes, and then my consultant went on holiday, and then, only then did they even talk about options for treatment. I'm 38 – they know I have time working against me! Finally, I am currently having my first cycle of IVF. (Lisa, 38)

Blood tests

All women have blood taken, and the following can be checked:

- Any time in your cycle – thyroid hormone levels, prolactin levels, androstendione (testosterone) levels.
- Day 2–3 of your cycle – tests taken for FSH, LH and oestradiol (a kind of oestrogen).
- Progesterone levels – taken in the second half of your cycle, seven days before your period is due. Sometimes serial progesterone levels will be taken, for example on days 21, 28 or 35.

Men may have blood tests depending on the results of their semen analysis, for example, FSH and LH levels, thyroid hormones and prolactin levels.

Infection screening

Both men and women should be screened for sexually transmitted diseases and other infections.

Women The test involves a speculum examination. Three swabs are taken, from the top of your vagina and inside your cervix. You may experience a pain like period pain as the swabs are taken. It is not abnormal to have a bit of bleeding or spotting after this examination.

You may also be asked to give a urine sample, taken mid-stream.

Men Urethral swab – a swab that looks like a long cottonbud, is inserted into the tip of your urethra (hole in the top of your penis) to check for infection.

You may also be asked to give a urine sample.

Ultrasound

Ultrasound works by sending sound waves into the body and waiting for them to be reflected (bounce back) to the machine. The machine then makes a 'picture' of your internal organs. Most women will have an ultrasound scan as part of their investigations. You can ask the ultrasonographer (person carrying out the ultrasound) to show you the screen and describe what they are seeing. Ultrasound scans take about five to ten minutes.

Transabdominal You will need a full bladder so you should drink lots of fluids in the few hours before the examination and not go to the toilet. You lie on your back with your abdomen exposed. Gel is placed on your lower abdomen and then a probe is moved over your tummy to look at your organs. Sometimes the ultrasonographer will have to push on your tummy with the probe – it shouldn't hurt but it may be a bit uncomfortable as you will have a full bladder.

Transvaginal Here a smaller probe is inserted into the vagina. You will be asked to empty your bladder before the test. The probe looks like a long tampon, the tip of which is inserted into the vagina. The probe is covered with a condom and lubricated with gel to ease insertion into the vagina, though this may feel cold. The reproductive organs can be examined in greater detail than in a transabdominal scan.

You may find this examination uncomfortable, but it shouldn't be painful. As with speculum examinations the more relaxed you are, the easier it will be.

Men may also have ultrasound scans:

Scrotal Gel is placed on the scrotum and a small probe moved over the scrotum to obtain pictures of the testes and tubes. This is a good method of discovering, for example, testicular masses, cysts and varicoceles.

Transrectal You will be asked to lie on your side with your knees pulled up to your chest. A small probe, covered with a condom and gel, is inserted into your back passage to look at the prostate gland and other structures in the genitalia.

Tests for women

Tests for ovulation

Self-testing Body basal temperature, cervical mucus testing and over the counter kits – see Chapter 3, How to increase your fertility.

Blood test As described above, a blood test in the second half of your cycle can tell doctors whether or not you have ovulated.

Ultrasound Serial transvaginal ultrasounds can be used to check for ovulation. From just before ovulation is expected ultrasound scans are carried out very regularly, as much as every day or every other day. Using transvaginal ultrasound, follicles can be tracked as they develop in the ovary. One will grow larger than the others. After ovulation the follicle changes in appearance and develops into the corpus luteum. If this is seen, then ovulation has occurred. This procedure is time-consuming as it involves regular trips to the ultrasound department of your clinic or hospital.

'Immunobead' test

This tests for the presence of anti-sperm antibodies within the woman. A blood sample is taken from the woman and the man produces a semen sample. The blood and semen are mixed together. The sperm are then examined under a microscope to see if they have been affected by any antibodies in the woman's blood.

Post-coital test

Also called the Sims-Huhner test, this is used to assess the cervical mucus after sexual intercourse, to determine whether it is hostile to sperm, and to see how many sperm are penetrating the mucus to enter the uterus via the cervix. Although it does not replace semen analysis, it can be used to test sperm if your male partner cannot give a sample. The test is controversial as it is unreliable. Studies have shown that the only reproducible result from post-coital testing is the number of sperm seen in the mucus.

Around ovulation oestrogen acts on the cervical mucus to make it thin to allow sperm to pass through. If the test is not performed around the time of ovulation it will not be accurate. Therefore you will have to assess when you are ovulating, using one of the methods described in the earlier chapter or by regular ultrasounds. The test must be carried out one or two days around the time of ovulation, between four and ten hours after sexual intercourse.

Have sex as normal but do not use any contraception or lubricants. Do not douche yourself or have a bath during or after intercourse as they could affect the results. You may have a shower.

Once at the doctor's you will be examined with a speculum; the doctor will remove a small sample of mucus from your cervix to be examined. You can then return to normal activities.

The most common reason for poor results is incorrect timing. Infection and previous surgery to the cervix such as laser cone biopsy for an abnormal smear can also affect results.

Hysterosalpingography (HSG)

This checks if your tubes are open. A harmless dye is put into the uterus, and X-rays are then taken as the dye moves through the uterus and into the fallopian tubes, allowing the doctor to look for any blockages or other problems. The ovaries cannot be seen with this procedure as they do not show up on X-rays. You are awake during the test. The test needs to be performed in the first ten days of your menstrual cycle but after your period has stopped.

It is important that there is no possibility of an early pregnancy when the test is performed as the dye may push a fertilized egg back into the tubes (increasing the risk of an ectopic pregnancy). Therefore you should not have any unprotected sex (though you can use a condom or diaphragm) from the time your period starts until after the test.

The dye used in the procedure can bring on cramps similar to period pain; you may want to take some painkillers such as paracetamol or ibuprofen an hour or so before the test and afterwards. You can return to your normal activities straightaway. It is normal to have some light bleeding or spotting for a day or two after the test. Once the test is performed you can attempt to become pregnant in that cycle.

What are the risks?

- A small risk from the radiation involved in taking X-rays.
- Infection may occur as an instrument (the catheter) is passed into the uterus. The doctors will perform this test using sterile techniques to reduce this risk. However, if after the test you have discharge with an offensive smell or have a temperature, you should see your doctor, as you may need antibiotics.
- If you have a very early pregnancy there is a risk the dye may push the fertilized egg back into the tubes.
- If you are allergic to shellfish or iodine you may have a reaction to the dye, which contains iodine – your doctor should ask but do say if you have any allergies.

There have been reports that HSG actually increases fertility. This may be due to the dye opening and straightening the fallopian tubes or affecting the cervical mucus.

Hysterosalpingo-contrast sonography (HyCoSy)

This is similar to hysterosalpingography. It is also used to check the patency of the tubes and to look at the cavity of the uterus to see if it is distorted, for example by fibroids. It is a non-invasive procedure done while you are awake. Harmless contrast dye is used to fill the uterus and tubes but instead of taking X-rays, ultrasound, generally transvaginal, is used to visualize the dye. The contrast dye used does not contain iodine and so this test can be performed in women allergic to iodine or shellfish. As no X-rays are used, there is no risk from radiation. The ovaries can be seen during the investigation as ultrasound is used.

As with HSG the insertion of the dye can cause a fertilized egg to be pushed back into the tubes. Therefore the test must be carried out in the first ten days of your cycle but after you have finished bleeding. You should not have unprotected sex from when you start bleeding until after the test.

You will be asked to empty your bladder before the procedure. A speculum is inserted into the vagina and a small catheter (tube) inserted into your cervix through which the contrast dye is inserted into the cavity. At the same time a transvaginal ultrasound probe will be inserted into the vagina and used to look at the flow of fluid through the uterus and tubes to check if they are open.

As with HSG, HyCoSy can bring on period pain-like cramps so you may want to take some painkillers about an hour before the procedure and afterwards. You can return to your normal activities straight after the test. It is normal to have some light vaginal bleeding after the test. Once the procedure is complete you can then try to get pregnant in the rest of that cycle.

What are the risks?

- Infection – if you develop an offensive smelling discharge or a fever please see a doctor, as you may need antibiotics.
- And as mentioned above, there is a risk of pushing a fertilized egg back into the tubes. Therefore the procedure is only carried out at a time in the cycle when there is no risk of pregnancy.

Hysteroscopy

This procedure allows your doctor to see inside your womb. It is used to look for fibroids or polyps and samples can be taken from the lining of the womb. The procedure takes about 10–15 minutes. Local or general anaesthetic may be used so you may be awake or asleep during the procedure depending on the facilities at your clinic, your own preferences and those of your doctor and anaesthetist which would take into account any other difficulties.

Your doctors will examine you and then insert a speculum; a small tube is then passed through the cervix and into the uterus. This tube is called a 'hysteroscope' and contains a small telescope which is hooked up to a television monitor allowing the doctor to see inside the womb. If you are awake you can ask to be shown the procedure on the television monitor.

Either gas or fluid, both harmless, is then run into the womb to make it expand so the doctor can see inside the cavity. The doctor then looks all around the cavity and ostia (where the fallopian tubes open into the uterus). Photos can be taken. If appropriate a sample of the lining of the womb may be taken, an endometrial biopsy. If taken at the appropriate time in the menstrual cycle, the sample can be analysed to see if the lining is developing as needed to allow implantation to occur.

It is normal to have a small amount of bleeding in the first few days after the procedure. You may also have period-like pains after the procedure and can take painkillers if you need them.

What are the risks?

- Bleeding – a small amount of bleeding is normal. If, as rarely occurs, your bleeding becomes very heavy you should return to the hospital immediately. If it is out of hours, please attend your local hospital emergency department.

- Infection – the procedure is carried out using sterile techniques but if you develop an offensive smelling discharge or get a fever you should see a doctor as you may need antibiotics.
- Perforation – there is a small risk that the hysteroscope causes a small tear in the wall of the uterus. This may need no treatment, but your doctor may ask you to stay in hospital overnight to observe for bleeding or infection. Rarely a tear will need to be repaired surgically.
- Fluid overload – fluid is inserted into the cavity of the uterus in order for a good view to be obtained. Your doctor will measure how much fluid is absorbed by your body; occasionally a large amount of fluid is absorbed. If this is the case you may be asked to stay in hospital overnight and have a blood test.

Laparoscopy and dye test

Also known as the 'lap and dye' test. A laparoscopy is keyhole surgery and is performed under a general anaesthetic. In the majority of cases you will be in hospital only for a day. Laparoscopy involves putting a telescope into the tummy and looking at the reproductive organs to see if there are any problems such as fibroids or endometriosis. It can be combined with hysteroscopy to look at the inside of the uterus.

A small cut (about 1–2cm) is made either in or just below the tummy button. The laparoscope (telescopic camera) is inserted through this cut. It is linked to a television monitor so the doctor can see your organs. Photos can be taken. Gas is passed into the tummy so it expands and the doctors can get a good view of the organs. Another cut may be made in your lower tummy, just above the pubic hair line. Depending on what is seen sometimes two other cuts may be made, one on each side of your lower tummy, also for surgical instruments. All of these cuts are small – about 1–2cm. If appropriate, biopsies can be taken.

Occasionally an even finer telescope is inserted through the openings of the fallopian tubes to look for an obstruction of the tubes from the inside – this is called falloscopy.

The 'and dye' part of the procedure involves inserting dye into the uterus through the cervix via a catheter and watching to see if the dye comes out of the tubes – if it does then the tubes must be open. Sometimes treatment is carried out during laparoscopy such as that for endometriosis (see Chapter 7, Medical and surgical treatment). A lap and dye procedure takes about 30–45 minutes.

You may need a few days off work to recover from the operation and may have some bloating after the procedure due to the gas used to inflate your tummy. This can also cause pain in your shoulders. The pain should pass within a week, and meanwhile painkillers may be helpful. Peppermint water may also help with the feeling of bloating. You may have some light vaginal bleeding.

The cuts may be sore; they should be kept dry for two days and then any plasters can be removed. You can then wash the wounds, with water only, but be sure to dry them carefully after washing. Do not use any creams or powders on the cuts. If stitches are used, they will generally dissolve on their own; you will be told if this is not the case and they need to be removed.

Some women find that a laparoscopy makes their next period start earlier than expected.

What are the risks?

- Bleeding – if large amounts of bleeding develop in the operation the surgeons may decide to make a larger cut (laparotomy) to give them better access to stop the bleeding.
- Infection – you will need to see a doctor if you develop redness around your cuts, fluid or pus oozing from the cuts, a fever or lots of pain.
- Damage to organs – this rarely occurs but there is a risk of damaging one of the organs during the procedure. If this occurs, as with bleeding, the surgeons may have to perform a laparotomy (larger cut) to repair any damage.

Tests for men

Semen analysis

Men will need to have had their sperm and semen analysed. For more information, see Chapter 5, Male causes of subfertility.

Testicular biopsy

This involves taking a small sample (biopsy) of the testis, to see if any sperm are being produced. It can be combined with sperm retrieval or harvesting procedures, and any sperm seen in the biopsy can be frozen for use in assisted reproduction (see Chapter 8, Assisted conception techniques and ethical issues).

The test is generally performed under local anaesthetic. You are awake for procedures that involve local anaesthetic, though sometimes a mild sedative is given to make you a little sleepy. You will feel the local anaesthetic being injected, a sharp, burning sensation, but after this you should feel no pain. You will still feel touch and pressure as

Having an anaesthetic

- For any procedure that involves a general anaesthetic, you will be asked to come into hospital a few weeks before the operation to be seen in a pre-assessment clinic. At this consultation a doctor or nurse will check that you are fit for the anaesthetic and operation and any necessary blood tests will be taken.
- You must not eat or drink for six hours prior to the operation.
- If you take medication please tell the nurse in the pre-assessment clinic and they will tell you whether or not they should be taken. Tablets should be taken with the minimum amount of water necessary.
- You will see both the anaesthetist and surgeon before the procedure, and they will explain what will happen to you. The surgeon will explain the risks and benefits of the procedure and you will be asked to sign a consent form.
- After the procedure you will be woken up in the recovery room and then will be taken back to your ward.
- If you are a 'day case' you will stay on the ward for a few hours and will be discharged once you have eaten and drunk and have passed urine.
- You will need to be accompanied home and should not be alone for the first 24 hours after the procedure.
- It is recommended that you do not drive, drink alcohol or operate machinery for 24 hours.

the doctor carries out the procedure but it should not be painful. If a sedative is also used you will need to be accompanied home.

There may be soreness in your testicles and/or bruises on your scrotum for a few days. Wearing tight, supportive underwear (not normally recommended in those with fertility problems) for a few days can help with the discomfort. It is advisable not to have sex for about a week or two after a biopsy.

Vasography

Vasography is used to assess the patency of the vas deferens (tubes that connect and carry the sperm from the epididymis to the urethra). It involves the injection of a contrast dye into the vas deferens to see if there is any obstruction. If contrast dye is also injected into the seminal vesicles (glands that produce seminal fluid) it is termed a vesiculogram.

7

Medical and surgical treatment

Medical treatment

Medical treatment takes a number of forms. In women, medications can be used to induce the production of eggs; and in men, they can be used for example to improve the sperm count or treat erectile dysfunction. The drug names used below are the generic names; often the same drug will have a different name if it is made by a different company. If you look at the active ingredient list of your medication, you should find one of the names below.

Medications for women

Ovulation induction

Ovulation induction aims to produce eggs in a cycle. Not all women are suitable, but it can be used for conditions such as hypogonadotrophic hypogonadism, stress, polycystic ovarian syndrome (PCOS) and idiopathic causes. The response to the treatment can be measured by whether your cycle restarts, blood or urine tests, or ultrasound scanning. Various medications are used:

Clomifene citrate

Clomifene is an 'anti-oestrogen'; it acts to convince the body that levels of oestrogen are low, causing the brain to produce more FSH, which in turn results in more follicles developing in the ovary. In this way, it kickstarts the normal cycle of egg production. Clomifene can affect other organs; your cervical mucus may not become thin, or the endometrium may not develop for implantation.

It is most commonly used in polycystic ovarian syndrome. About 70 per cent of women with PCOS taking clomifene will start ovulating. Ovulation does not automatically mean that pregnancy will occur straightaway, but after six months of clomifene treatment the conception rate is about 50 per cent.

How do I take it? Clomifene is taken orally, at home, for five days, starting on day 2–5 of your cycle. Ovulation should occur five to ten days after your last dose of clomifene. Therefore, a week after you take your last dose you should start having regular sex. If you are not having cycles, your doctor may induce a period with progesterone so you can start taking clomifene.

You may also be given one injection of human chorionic gonadotrophin (HCG) in the middle of your cycle. The HCG simulates the body's natural surge of LH so ovulation can occur.

What are the side effects? As with any drug that stimulates the production of follicles, there is a small risk of ovarian hyperstimulation syndrome (see next chapter). You may have ultrasounds to monitor the number of follicles developing in the ovaries.

Other possible side effects may be symptoms of the menopause such as hot flushes; and abdominal pain and nausea. There is a risk of multiple pregnancy – about 10 per cent of those taking clomifene will have twins.

Gonadotrophins – Follicle stimulating hormone (FSH)

FSH is used for women with hypothalamic-pituitary causes of anovulation, or PCOS. It acts to produce follicles in the ovary, and so induce ovulation. As with clomifene, an injection of HCG may also be needed. Some studies have shown that FSH injections can increase fertility to a level even higher than couples without problems.

How do I take it? FSH is given by injection, either under the skin or into a muscle. You will be shown how to inject the medication and safely dispose of any needles. You could do it yourself or get your partner to help by giving you the injections.

You will be monitored by transvaginal ultrasound scans to see how many follicles are being produced, and once the follicles are of a certain size, you will be asked to start having regular sex.

What are the side effects? Abdominal pain, breast tenderness and reaction at the site of injections. The most serious side effect is ovarian hyperstimulation syndrome (see next chapter). There is also a high rate of multiple pregnancy.

Gonadotrophin releasing hormone (GnRH)

GnRH analogues are used in women with hypothalamic causes of anovulation such as that related to body weight. They work by stopping your cycles. You will then be given FSH injections to create follicles followed by one shot of HCG to stimulate ovulation. This gives the best control over the induction of ovulation. GnRH analogues can increase fertility to the same levels as the general population.

How do I take it? Nasal spray, or a small pump is worn on your arm, which releases pulses of GnRH under the skin (via a tiny needle) every 90 minutes.

What are the side effects? There may be reactions around the site of injection. Symptoms of the menopause are also possible – hot flushes, mood swings, depression, loss of libido, vaginal dryness, lethargy and headaches.

Medications for men

Hormone treatments

Clomifene may be used to correct hormone imbalances and improve the quantity and quality of sperm. There is little evidence to support this theory at present.

Gonadotrophins Injections of FSH can be used in hypogonadotrophin hypogonadism.

Steroids

Some doctors may use steroids to treat men with anti-sperm antibodies. This treatment is controversial as the effects of anti-sperm antibodies on fertility are not yet known. Steroids are very potent drugs with many side effects such as stomach ulcers and osteoporosis.

Drugs for sexual dysfunction

There are various medications for erectile dysfunction. Other medications can be used, for example, to strengthen the neck of the bladder to prevent retrograde ejaculation. It is important you inform your doctor that you are also trying to conceive, as some medications may have an adverse effect on fertility.

Surgical treatment

There are various surgical options for the treatment of subfertility, for both men and women, depending on the cause of the subfertility.

Surgical treatments for women

Surgical ovarian induction

Surgical induction can be used in women with PCOS. Success rates are similar to those of medical ovulation with FSH injections. It is thought to work by decreasing the amount of androgens (testosterones) produced by the ovary. The procedure is called ovarian diathermy or 'drilling', and is a type of keyhole (laparoscopic) surgery performed under general anaesthetic. About six holes are made in the ovary either using diathermy (heat), or laser.

The risk of ovarian hyperstimulation or multiple pregnancy with drilling is lower than with medical induction. Apart from the risks of the laparoscopy (see Chapter 6, Diagnostic tests), there is a risk that too much of the ovary is destroyed, potentially resulting in premature menopause.

Transcervical tubal cannulation

Tubal cannulation aims to unblock any blocked tubes. It generally involves hysterosalpingography (see Chapter 6, Diagnostic tests) and is performed on an outpatient basis. Radio-opaque dye is inserted through a catheter in the cervix and then X-rays are taken. A guide wire is passed into the uterus and fallopian tubes to dislodge any debris that may be blocking the tube. The dye should then be seen on x-ray spilling out of the now unblocked tube. The procedure takes about 30 minutes.

Some clinics offer 'balloon tubuloplasty' – here a balloon is inserted into the tube and then blown up to dislodge any blockages.

Hysteroscopy

A hysteroscopy aimed at treating a problem, as opposed to a diagnostic hysteroscopy, is always performed under general anaesthetic. Hysteroscopy can be used to treat problems within the cavity of the womb such as intrauterine fibroids, intrauterine adhesions or a septum.

For more information on this procedure, see Chapter 6, Diagnostic tests.

Laparoscopy/laparotomy

Surgery can be carried out via laparoscopy (keyhole surgery) or laparotomy (open surgery where a larger cut is made in the abdomen) under general anaesthetic. Lasers can be used as well as more traditional surgical tools. (See Chapter 6, Diagnostic tests.) Various procedures can be used to treat tubal subfertility during the operation. There may be a higher rate of ectopic pregnancy (pregnancy outside the womb) after these procedures:

- *Fimbrioplasty* reconstructs a damaged end to the fallopian tube.
- *Tubal reanastomosis* is the term used for the reversal of female sterilization. In sterilization the tubes are tied (tubal ligation); this operation aims to reconnect and open them.
- *Neosalingostomy* means opening a blocked fallopian tube.
- *Salpingolysis* means the removal of adhesions from a fallopian tube.
- *Salpingectomy* means the removal of a fallopian tube, carried out when the tube is irreversibly damaged or contains collections of pus and fluid from an infection. In these situations, removing the tube can increase the success rate of IVF.

Surgery can also be carried out to treat other problems during laparoscopy/laparotomy, such as removing adhesions or deposits of endometriosis or removing fibroids.

Surgical treatments for men

Surgery for obstructive azoospermia

Obstructive azoospermia is a condition in which sperm are produced in the testis but are prevented from being released in the ejaculate due to a blockage in one of the connecting tubes.

Vasovavostomy

This procedure involves removing the blocked portion of a tube. It is used to reverse vasectomies (male sterilization) and can result in about 80 per cent of men having sperm in their ejaculate again.

Vasoepididymostomy

In this procedure the section of the vas deferens just before any blockage is attached directly to the epididymis to allow sperm to pass through, avoiding any blockage in between. Men are asked to give semen samples on a regular basis after the procedure, approximately every three months. This is to check that scar tissue has not formed, reblocking the tubes and again preventing sperm from entering the ejaculate.

Success rates depend on the length of time the blockage has been present – if it has been there for a long time, your body may have stopped producing sperm or may start to produce anti-sperm antibodies, which may cause problems. Any sperm obtained during the procedure can be frozen and stored for future use in assisted reproduction.

Varicocelectomy

This is an operation to remove a varicocele. An alternative is embolization, where a clot is sent into the varicocele so it no longer has a blood supply.

Recent studies suggest there is little evidence that varicocelectomy improves pregnancy rates; however, it may improve the quality of sperm.

Sperm retrieval

Sperm retrieval or sperm harvesting is when sperm are extracted from the testes or tubes for use in assisted reproductive techniques. The technique used will depend on the cause of your low sperm count. If you have a low sperm count due to a blockage, the techniques used will be MESE, PESA or TESA (all described below); if you have a low sperm count not related to obstruction, the techniques available are TESE or TESA (see below). These techniques can also be used in ejaculatory failure.

In all the situations described below, sperm can be used straightaway if the procedure has been timed correctly with ovulation. Any extra sperm can be frozen and stored for future use to prevent you having to have multiple procedures to harvest sperm.

All the following procedures can be carried out under local anaesthetic, with or without sedation, or under a general anaesthetic. Recovery from the procedure itself is quick, generally within a day or so. In all situations you may be sore and swollen for a few days afterwards; this may be helped by painkillers and tight supportive underwear. Risks associated with these techniques are bleeding and infection.

Microsurgical epididymal sperm extraction/aspiration (MESE)

A small incision is made in the skin of the scrotum to find the epididymis (tube where sperm are stored and mature). The epididymis contains many small tubes; some of these are opened and the fluid inside collected and examined for sperm. This technique is invasive as it involves cutting the skin. However, it has a high success rate for finding sperm.

Percutaneous epididymal sperm aspiration (PESA)

A needle is inserted into the epididymis to withdraw some fluid which is examined under a microscope for sperm. The procedure is less invasive than MESE. However, as no incision is made in the skin, the doctor cannot see into the epididymis; it is less accurate than MESE so fewer sperm may be found. Also the risk of bruising is greater than with MESE.

Testicular sperm extraction from a testicular biopsy (TESE)

A small incision is made in the skin, through which a very small sample (biopsy) of the testis itself is taken. As with MESE, it is an invasive procedure. In the lab the sample of testicular tissue is divided into smaller pieces which are then examined to see if any sperm can be retrieved from the seminiferous tubules, where they are made within the testes.

Testicular sperm aspiration (TESA, also called testicular FNA)

A needle is inserted through a small cut in the skin and used to obtain a sample of testicular tissue. The retrieval rates may be lower than with TESE as less tissue is obtained.

Vas deferens sperm aspiration

A needle is inserted into the vas deferens and fluid withdrawn and examined for sperm. The procedure is non-invasive as no incision is made and so has a quick recovery time. The epididymis may be massaged to try to bring more sperm into the vas deferens. The sperm obtained from the vas are generally more mature than those obtained from the epididymis or testis.

8

Assisted conception techniques and ethical issues

Assisted conception, or assisted reproductive techniques, aims to re-create the natural process of conception. Eggs can be produced naturally or with stimulated cycles, the sperm is prepared by sperm washing and then the procedures aim to bring the sperm and egg together to aid fertilization. In any of the techniques, the chances of success decrease with increasing maternal age.

Preparation of an egg: Superovulation vs natural cycles

Superovulation

Superovulation is a process in which medication is given to produce several follicles without one follicle becoming dominant, so that many eggs are produced. The more eggs you produce, the greater the chance that one of those eggs will be fertilized by sperm to produce a zygote and eventually a baby. However, producing too many eggs carries a risk of hyperstimulation syndrome and multiple pregnancy.

> The injections – that was the bit I felt was hardest on me and my husband felt was hardest on him. I was the one having the injections every day, with bruises all over me, terrible headaches and nausea and still having to go to work every day. He didn't have to go through any of it! Of course, he felt his lot was just as bad, I made him give me the injections every night and he said he hated being the one actually giving me the injections he knew I hated! The mood swings meant he never knew how I was going to be, when I would freak out, though at the time I never felt I was being unreasonable, no matter what the hysterical tears were about! Who had it harder, me, who had to take the drugs, or him who had to live with the effects of them? Once our child was born, it all became worth it. (Seema, 36)

Ovulation is induced as described in Chapter 7, Medical and surgical treatment. Either injections of gonadotrophins (FSH) alone or GnRH analogues or antagonists with gonadotrophins are used.

For intrauterine insemination (IUI) you are aiming for up to three eggs, from three mature follicles. If too many eggs are produced, increasing the chances of a multiple pregnancy of a number that cannot be supported by the body, your cycle may be cancelled. For in vitro fertilization (IVF) and intracytoplasmic sperm injection (ICSI), you need more eggs as they are collected and then put back into you after being fertilized. Here we are aiming for more eggs, at least four or five. The risk of grand multiple pregnancy is not an issue in these circumstances at this point because not all the embryos produced are transferred back to the womb.

From about day 9 of your superovulatory cycle you will start to have regular transvaginal ultrasounds to measure how many follicles there are and how they are developing. You may also be given blood tests to determine follicular development. The eggs themselves cannot be seen but the size of the follicles corresponds to the maturity of the eggs. Once the follicles have reached a diameter of about 18mm, you will be asked to give yourself an injection of human chorionic gonadotrophin (HCG). This simulates the rise in LH in the natural menstrual cycle, resulting in the final stage of maturation of the eggs before ovulation.

If it is felt that too many follicles are developing, thus putting you at risk of ovarian hyperstimulation syndrome (described below), the cycle will be stopped.

What are the risks?

Ovarian hyperstimulation syndrome (OHSS) This is the most serious risk of any superovulation treatment and occurs if the body is very sensitive to the gonadotrophin injections, resulting in a very large number of follicles in the ovaries.

Why the condition occurs is not yet known. It is thought the high levels of oestrogen produced by the many follicles can result in changes to the 'leakiness' of blood vessels, allowing fluid to accumulate where it should not, for example in the lungs or abdomen. There is also an increased risk of blood clots developing.

Symptoms can occur at any time but tend to occur about a week after your medications have finished. They include feeling generally unwell, abdominal pain, swelling in the abdomen, shortness of breath, ankle swelling, nausea and vomiting, either constipation or diarrhoea, dark concentrated urine or passing very little urine irregularly, chest pain or pain in your calves.

If you develop any of the above symptoms you must go to your doctor (if out of hours, to your local emergency department). It is important your doctors are aware of your symptoms and that you are checked over, even if you have a mild case, as ovarian hyperstimulation syndrome is a serious condition. If you are in the early phase of a cycle, then further treatment in this cycle may be stopped.

In mild cases, you will be told to return for check-ups regularly and to return if symptoms worsen. Drink lots of water. In more severe cases, you will be admitted to hospital, and given medication to prevent blood clots, as well as regular blood tests and occasionally fluids through a drip. If you have a lot of fluid collected in your abdomen or are very short of breath, the doctors may drain the fluid from your tummy or chest to relieve the symptoms.

Doctors try to prevent OHSS by tailoring dosages of drugs to each patient and by monitoring how many follicles are developing by ultrasound. If too many follicles are developing, your treatment cycle may be stopped. Those at an increased risk of OHSS include women under 30 and women with PCOS. Women in at-risk groups for developing OHSS will be monitored carefully and may not be given the HCG injection to try and prevent the development of OHSS.

Multiple pregnancy While you are trying to have a baby, it is understandable that the thought of having two or three at once may actually be desirable. However, the more foetuses you carry at one time, the greater the risks to both you and the foetuses. The risks are greatest when carrying three or more foetuses. There is an increased risk of cerebral palsy and of lower birth weights and prematurity, with all their related problems and higher death and disability rates.

Although we aim for three eggs to be produced in IUI and limit the number of embryos transferred back into the womb during IVF there is still a risk of multiple pregnancy. After all, if you produce more eggs, there is an increased chance of you getting pregnant, and that includes getting pregnant naturally. Alternatively, as with natural conception an embryo could divide naturally to form a multiple pregnancy.

Natural cycles

A natural cycle is one where no medication is given. The development of a follicle during your normal menstrual cycle is tracked using transvaginal ultrasound. Around the time of ovulation IUI can then be performed, or the egg collected for use in other techniques. It cannot be used if the tubes are blocked or if you are not ovulating regularly. As no medication is used there are no risks or side effects. Natural cycle treatments are also significantly cheaper than treatment with stimulated cycles as the cost of the medications is removed. However, fewer eggs are produced, generally one egg per cycle, occasionally two, and therefore the chances of conception may be lower. Using IVF, after three to four treatments, the pregnancy rates between natural and stimulated cycles are similar. Not all fertility centres offer natural cycles.

It may be that you could have a combination of the two forms of treatment, using low-dose medications to induce ovulation.

Preparation of sperm

In assisted reproduction the sperm are obtained from a sample of semen. For more information on how to produce your sample of semen, see the semen analysis section in Chapter 5, Male causes of subfertility. The sperm sample may have to be produced within a certain timeframe to coincide with any other procedures that are taking place, or be frozen in advance.

The semen is then 'washed' to remove any dead sperm, unwanted cells or substances that may interfere with fertility. Semen contains prostaglandins; if they are not removed they can cause contractions of the uterus similar to period pain. Sperm can also be washed to decrease the risk of passing on an infection, such as HIV. Ordinarily only sperm and not the rest of the contents of the semen enter the uterus; in assisted conception the aim is to try and simulate nature as much as possible and therefore only the sperm are needed.

Sperm washing involves diluting and spinning the semen at a very high speed in a centrifuge. This divides the sperm from the semen and allows the doctor to select the best sperm for use in treatment. The sperm are then put in a nutrient-rich fluid that enables sperm maturation to occur.

After sperm washing you will have a sample of sperm that are the healthiest and are the most likely to result in fertilization for use in assisted reproduction.

Artificial insemination

Artificial insemination describes any situation in which the sperm is placed in the woman by means other than during sexual intercourse. The advantage is that this is the closest to natural conception of all the assisted reproductive techniques. It's relatively simple and cheap and causes the least stress on the woman's body.

> IUI was our first actual treatment and we were convinced it was going to work, which it did, in the end. I was convinced that once the doctors stepped in I would get pregnant on the first try, after all that is what doctors do, don't they, fix the problem? It was an odd sensation really – instead of working out my most fertile time and then hounding my poor partner for regular sex, it was all worked out by scan and then the actual procedure, which used to be sex at home, done for us by him giving a sample and then the doctors putting it inside me. Before we had always made love thinking that it would create a baby. I felt that the love part had been taken away, that it had become something clinical. Of course now I realize that that was not the case, that we were still making a baby out of love, just that we needed a bit of help! (Rachel, 34)

Intrauterine insemination

Intrauterine insemination (IUI) involves placing sperm directly into the uterus at the most fertile point in the cycle to increase the likelihood of conception, i.e. at ovulation. It bypasses a few steps in natural conception such as male ejaculation and sperm swimming through the cervical mucus. It gives the sperm a head start on the way to fertilizing an egg. The aim is that once in the uterus, the sperm will swim to the tubes, fertilize an egg and result in a pregnancy as normal.

IUI is generally the first form of treatment in unexplained subfertility. It can be used in male subfertility – where there is a mild or low sperm count, sperm that don't swim well or are abnormal in form, antisperm antibodies, or some kind of failure of ejaculation. IUI can also be used when medical induction of ovulation has failed or where there are cervical problems.

A significant advantage of IUI is that it causes the least disruption to the woman's cycle, especially if natural cycles are used. This means that you may be able to tolerate more cycles. Either superovulatory or natural cycle ovulation can be used, depending on your own preference and the cause of your fertility problems.

Some clinics may offer 'double IUI', where two inseminations are given during one menstrual cycle. There is currently no evidence to suggest that double insemination increases pregnancy rates when compared to single insemination.

What it involves

The procedure takes place around the time of ovulation – monitored by ultrasound. You will be examined with a speculum. A very small, soft tube is inserted through your cervix and about 0.25ml of prepared sperm (not semen, just the sperm) is injected through the cervix into the uterus.

You may want to take some painkillers about an hour before the procedure as the act of passing the tube into the cervix can cause some discomfort. Some women may experience mild cramps for a few hours after the procedure, which takes about five minutes. You will then be able to return to your normal activities straightaway. You can have sex throughout your cycle using IUI, even shortly after the procedure. A pregnancy test can be performed from 14 days after the insemination has taken place.

What are the chances of success?

The chances of becoming pregnant depend on the cause of the subfertility, whether donated sperm/eggs, natural or stimulated cycles were used, and will also vary between clinics. The success rate is generally between 10 and 20 per cent. Generally, the chances of success are increased if mild ovarian stimulation is used.

Most clinics will try IUI for three to six cycles. The majority of couples who will conceive using IUI do so within six cycles; if there has been no success after this point, your doctor may advise you to try a different treatment, such as IVF.

Intratubal insemination

In intratubal insemination (ITI), also known as fallopian sperm perfusion, the sperm are placed directly into the fallopian tube. Natural or superovulatory cycles can be used and the timing is as for IUI. The procedure is very similar to IUI but an ultrasound probe is used to place the sperm in, or at the entrance to, the fallopian tube. ITI currently has higher pregnancy rates than IUI for unexplained subfertility.

Intraperitoneal insemination (IPI)

Intraperitoneal insemination involves placing the sperm, not through the cervix into the uterus, but into the pelvis, near the open ends of the fallopian tubes. Again, chances of pregnancy are increased if the procedure is carried out around the time of ovulation. The procedure is carried out under ultrasound guidance: a speculum is inserted into the vagina and then a small needle passed through the top of the vagina into the pelvis. Using the ultrasound as guide, the doctor will try and place the sperm, via the needle, into the pelvis near the opening of the fallopian tube so the sperm will travel down the tube to meet and hopefully fertilize an egg. This is not routinely used.

Intracervical insemination (ICI)

In intracervical insemination, the sperm are placed into, but not through, the cervix. As with IUI, at the correct time in the cycle, a tube is inserted into, but not through, the cervix and the prepared sperm injected into the cervix. A cap like a diaphragm may then be put over the cervix for about eight hours to try and prevent the sperm from leaking out. You should rest for about 30 minutes after the procedure. This treatment can be used for those with ejaculatory problems but has not been shown to increase the chances of pregnancy for those with other causes of subfertility.

Intravaginal insemination (IVI)

Intravaginal or transvaginal insemination is a process that mimics the situation after sexual intercourse. It is used only if there is a problem with ejaculation or for surrogacy. Again, it has the best chances of success if timed to coincide with ovulation. In this procedure washed sperm or unprepared semen can be used. The semen is placed directly into the vagina and then it is advised that you rest for about 30 minutes. IVI can be done by the doctor but you could also carry out this procedure at home, calculating when you ovulate and inserting the sperm into the vagina using a clean syringe.

Procedures such as intracervical or intravaginal insemination are very cheap and simple. However, they are only likely to work in those whose only problem is ejaculatory failure. If there are any other factors to your subfertility but you are still suitable for insemination, IUI or ITI may be more appropriate.

Gamete intrafallopian transfer (GIFT)

Gamete intrafallopian transfer was first used in 1984. Eggs and sperm (both referred to as gametes) are collected and then placed in the fallopian tube. GIFT allows the process of fertilization to occur within the woman (in vivo), at the site where it occurs during natural conception. In GIFT the eggs do not have to be picked up by the end of the tube and the sperm do not have to swim through the female genital tract to reach an egg. Initially GIFT was thought of as a more natural option than IVF as the fertilization process occurs within the woman; however, it does involve a general anaesthetic and a surgical procedure (laparoscopy).

GIFT is used for couples who have tried IUI or other forms of artificial insemination without success. It can also be used in mild male subfertility, endometriosis or unexplained subfertility. For those who may have religious or other objections to fertilization occurring outside the body as in IVF, GIFT may be more acceptable.

The treatment requires natural or stimulated ovulation, egg retrieval and sperm preparation, and about 100,000–200,000 sperm are used. The transfer occurs during laparoscopy under general anaesthetic (for more information about laparoscopy, please see Chapter 6, Diagnostic tests). The eggs and sperm are placed in the fallopian tube through a small tube. About 25–30 per cent of women become pregnant in any cycle.

It is recommended that only three eggs are placed back in the tubes along with the sperm, or two in young women. However, GIFT is not regulated by the HFEA unless donor gametes are used and so clinics that are not licensed by the HFEA may offer to put back more than three eggs, which has an increased risk of grand multiple pregnancy.

In vitro fertilization (IVF)

In vitro fertilization is probably the most famous of all the assisted reproductive techniques. The first child to be born via IVF was born in 1978. Eggs and sperm are combined in a laboratory (in vitro literally means 'in glass', referring to the test tube or Petri dish in which fertilization occurs), the fertilized egg is then allowed to develop and is then put back in the womb. As the fertilization process occurs in the lab, this has been dubbed as creating 'test-tube babies'.

IVF can be used in women with blocked tubes, severe endometriosis, problems with ovulation or if a donor egg is used. It can be used in mild male subfertility, though the sperm still need to be able to fertilize an egg without assistance. It can also be used in unexplained subfertility or where IUI has failed.

IVF involves the following phases: ovulation, collection of the eggs, fertilization of the eggs by sperm and transferring the fertilized eggs back into the uterus.

Ovulation

This can occur naturally or with stimulated cycles to achieve superovulation. The more eggs that are produced the greater the number that can be collected, increasing the chances that some will be fertilized and then develop far enough to be transferred back into the uterus; some fertilized eggs could also be frozen for future use. The benefits of collecting many eggs has to be weighed up against the risk of hyperstimulation. If too many follicles are developing, your cycle may be stopped. Cycles may also be cancelled if too few follicles are developing.

Egg collection

During egg collection, the eggs are retrieved from the follicles. This is carried out under sedation or general anaesthetic and takes about 30 minutes. If you are having sedation you will be awake but sleepy, and should not be aware of any pain. Your partner may be allowed to stay with you.

Ultrasound is used to guide the doctor to the follicles. A small needle is inserted through the top of the vagina into the fluid filled follicles. The fluid is drawn up into a syringe and taken straight to the laboratory where it is examined under the microscope to see if it contains an egg. Not all follicles will contain an egg. As with all assisted reproduction techniques, timing is everything: eggs are only capable of being fertilized for a short time; too young or too mature and they may not be fertilized or develop normally. Each egg is graded for maturity to decide when it should be inseminated.

Your abdomen may feel a bit tender afterwards. You can take painkillers for any discomfort. You may also see some light bleeding, spotting or browny discharge for a few days. However, if you develop heavy bleeding, severe pain, a fever or offensive smelling discharge you will need to see your doctor.

Fertilization

The collected eggs are stored in an incubator, at body temperature, in a fluid that contains all the nutrients required for fertilization and early development. Each egg is inseminated with a sample of sperm. Approximately 12–24 hours later, the eggs are examined to see if fertilization has occurred. Normally about 60 per cent of eggs become fertilized. The fertilized egg divides into two cells and then further divisions occur, initially at approximately 24-hour intervals. By day 2 they are generally four cells and by day 3, six to eight cells. Eggs may not fertilize if there is a problem with the sperm or egg, or may become fertilized and then stop developing.

Embryo transfer

The procedure of embryo transfer is essentially the same as that used in IUI, but embryos are transferred into the uterus instead of sperm. The regulations regarding how many embryos can be transferred back into your womb may change in the near future. Currently two embryos can be transferred back in women under 40. This may be decreased to one embryo in the hope of reducing the number of multiple pregnancies; conversely this may also reduce the likelihood of a successful IVF cycle. Some centres only offer transfer of one embryo if you are under 35. Currently women over 40, who are using their own eggs, can have up to three embryos transferred. If donor eggs are used, currently only two embryos are transferred irrespective of the woman's age.

Generally, embryos are transferred back into the womb on day 2 or 3, when they are between four and eight cells in size. Some clinics offer blastocyst transfer, when the fertilized eggs are kept in culture for five to seven days. As they are then larger, this may allow the doctors to transfer back the embryos that have the best chance of survival. At present there is no evidence to suggest higher birth rates after transfer on day 5 when compared to transfer on day 2 to 3. The long-term effects of keeping embryos out of the womb for five days is not yet known.

In order for the embryos to implant, the lining of the womb needs to be thick, and the thickness of the endometrium is determined using ultrasound scan. If the endometrium is less than 5mm thick, the embryo is not likely to implant. Progesterone can be given to try and thicken the endometrium before transfer or the embryos can be frozen for use in future cycles.

As with IUI, a small tube is inserted through the cervix into the uterus and the embryos injected into womb where they will hopefully implant. Transfer is carried out under ultrasound guidance, so you see your embryos being put back into your womb. This ultrasound is a transabdominal, so you should drink lots of fluids in the few hours before the procedure so you have a full bladder to enable a better picture. Some people may experience mild cramps after the procedure, for which you can take painkillers. You are advised to rest for 20–30 minutes afterwards.

Progesterone support

After the embryos have been transferred back into your womb there is a waiting period to see whether or not they have implanted and you have become pregnant. If you have had natural cycle IVF, your body will be producing progesterone to help thicken the lining of the womb to prepare for implantation and support the embryo at this time. Those using stimulated cycles may not be producing as much progesterone and so may be given extra progesterone either until they have a positive pregnancy test or, if less lucky, start their period.

The progesterone can be taken as either oral tablets, injections or vaginal pessaries. Even if you are having a natural cycle, you may be advised to take progesterone. Side effects of progesterone include breast swelling and tenderness and nausea or vomiting.

About 12–14 days after your embryos have been transferred back inside your womb you can take your first pregnancy test, either a blood or a urine test. If the result is unclear, you may be asked to repeat a blood test after 48 hours.

> When you are trying naturally, each month you mourn for what might have been, but with IVF, when it doesn't work there was actually something real and physical to mourn. We had produced embryos, that were alive in the lab, I saw them, saw them being implanted in me and I couldn't keep them, nourish them, and so they died. I had something that was alive and when my period came I knew that they had died, I felt I had lost my child. (Gaby, 42)

> That two-week wait is the longest of your life. This time I know that fertilization took place, that we made an embryo. A live embryo was transferred back, will it stay there, will we be pregnant? (Jonathan, 37)

What are the chances of success?

Success is dependent on the cause of your subfertility, whether your own or donor egg or sperm were used and your age. For women under the age of 35, the chances of a live birth per cycle are approximately 20–25 per cent.

Your chances of success are increased if you have had a previous pregnancy, whether or not that pregnancy resulted in a live birth. If you have large collections in your fallopian tubes, surgical removal of the tubes (salpingectomy) increases success rates.

> Before I started IVF I felt that there was only one point in the month where I was either going to be pregnant or not. Of course

Risks of IVF

- Risks of the medications for superovulation as described above including ovarian hyperstimulation.
- Risk of any anaesthetic used.
- Multiple pregnancy – carries an increased risk of miscarriage, premature birth and maternal problems such as severe morning sickness or gestational diabetes.
- Miscarriage – this is the same as for any pregnancy: between 15 to 25 per cent of recognized pregnancies will miscarry. The true number may be higher than this but the women may not yet be aware they are pregnant. In the IVF situation you will always know you have had live embryos transferred back into you, and so will be aware that these have been lost if you do not become pregnant.
- Ectopic pregnancy – one that develops outside the womb, most commonly in the fallopian tubes. It is a potentially dangerous situation as the tube cannot stretch as the pregnancy grows, and if not treated can burst. Even though the embryos are transferred back into the uterus during IVF there is a chance that they will then travel and implant in the tubes. The risk of ectopic pregnancy in the general population is about 1 per cent; this increases in IVF pregnancies to 4–5 per cent.
- Low birth weight – IVF babies are more than two and a half times more likely to be born underweight than those conceived naturally. At present the reason for this is unknown. Being underweight at birth can cause various problems including problems with control of temperature and blood sugars.
- Congenital malformations – IVF babies appear to be 1–2 per cent more likely to have a malformation than those conceived naturally. The reason for this is also as yet unknown.

I thought about it constantly, probably most of the time I had sex I was wondering whether or not this time would be the magic time that got me pregnant, but there was only one time in the month when I would wonder if I actually was pregnant, the time around my period! Once I started IVF I felt that I could succeed or fail at every stage and so every stage brought about the whole range of emotions – how many eggs will I produce, how many will they collect, will they fertilize, will they develop, will they implant? At some point or other I felt that I have failed at every

> stage – instead of thinking how fantastic it was to collect four or six eggs, I would think that I wished I had produced more. For every egg that didn't fertilize or every embryo that didn't develop, I felt that we failed. When we had to stop our last cycle because we had no embryos to transfer back, it felt like the end of the world, that I went through all the physical discomfort for nothing. (Hatty, 39)

As with all aspects of fertility, IVF has greater success rates if you are not under or overweight, and if you and your partner do not smoke or consume too much alcohol or caffeine (see Chapter 3, How to increase your fertility).

The chances of success with IVF decrease with increasing maternal age from 20–25 per cent in those under 35 to approximately 10 per cent for women aged 39–40. Finally, different clinics will have different success rates. For more information on success rates, see Chapter 2, Starting your journey.

Storage of embryos

During IVF, you may produce more embryos than can legally be transferred back into you. The question then arises as to what should happen to any remaining embryos. You may want to store them for use in future cycles, either if a cycle is cancelled due to ovarian hyperstimulation, if no eggs are collected or if you do not want to go through superovulation and egg collection again. The cost of storing embryos may or may not be included in the price of your cycle.

Healthy, developing embryos are stored by freezing (cryopreservation). You and your partner sign a consent form to store the embryos for up to five years. At the time of writing, the Human Tissue and Embryos Bill is being discussed by a parliamentary expert committee. One of the recommendations of the Bill is that the storage time for embryos be increased to ten years. It is expected that a decision will be made by the end of 2007. Not all embryos may survive freezing and then thawing. Other options include donating your embryos to other couples or to research, or discarding the embryos.

Both you and your partner must consent to anything that happens to your embryos, from discarding them to using them in treatment. If one partner changes his/her mind and withdraws consent, for example if you split up, then neither party can use the embryos, which are then discarded.

Intracytoplasmic sperm injection (ICSI)

Intracytoplasmic sperm injection was first developed in 1992. It is a form of IVF in which the sperm are helped to fertilize an egg. As the quantity and/or the quality of the sperm used to inseminate the eggs in IVF falls, so does the number of eggs that become fertilized. The more irregular the sperm, the greater the risk of failure of fertilization.

ICSI is very similar to IVF – ovulation is induced and eggs are collected, the eggs are then fertilized and the resulting embryos are transferred back into the uterus with the hope of producing a pregnancy. Sperm can be obtained from a semen sample or using any of the sperm harvesting techniques described in Chapter 7, Medical and surgical treatment. The difference is the method of fertilization: each egg is not inseminated with thousands of sperm; the healthiest sperm are selected and a single sperm inserted through the outer shell of a mature egg, directly into the centre of the egg.

ICSI is used to treat male causes of subfertility that involve problems with either the number or the quality of the sperm. Therefore it can be used for those with low sperm counts for whatever reason, including obstructive causes, those with immunological problems or ejaculatory problems, or if IVF with traditional egg insemination has failed.

> My girlfriend told me a thousand times that it wasn't my fault, that this was our problem, that we would solve it together, I had begun to believe her. But that was just while we were having the investigations and waiting for treatment. Now that we were actually having ICSI, I felt awful again! If I made better sperm she wouldn't have to go through this, I was the one making her have the injections, the egg collection, the headaches, the watching, waiting and hoping. I really felt that I was putting her through all this pain, the one person that I never wanted to hurt, wanted to give her everything she wanted. It was only when she was pregnant and I saw the relief and happiness that it brought her that I realized that she wanted it as much as me, that it was that we wanted a child, not just me, and that we would have done anything to have one, the process seemed less important then. (Ali, 39)

Risks

Risks include those related to IVF as described above including the increased risk of low birth weight. There is also an increased risk of the foetus having a chromosomal abnormality (e.g. Down's syndrome) or other congenital abnormality. This is thought to be because sperm used in ICSI may be immature or abnormal and therefore more likely to have chromosomal abnormalities.

Chances of success

The chances of fertilization are approximately 60–70 per cent. However, fertilization is just one step in the pathway and does not necessarily mean that a pregnancy will occur. After fertilization, the chances of a pregnancy are the same as for a traditional IVF cycle.

Zygote intrafallopian transfer (ZIFT)

Zygote intrafallopian transfer is similar to both GIFT and IVF. Fertilization occurs in the laboratory but the developing fertilized eggs (zygotes) are transferred back into the fallopian tubes instead of the uterus. ZIFT can be used for all couples that are suitable for IVF and may have a further factor making it difficult to transfer the embryos into the uterus, for example, cervical stenosis. It cannot be used if you have blocked fallopian tubes. As it involves superovulation, egg retrieval, egg insemination with sperm for fertilization in the laboratory and then surgery to transfer the zygotes, it is considered to be a very invasive technique and is therefore only rarely used, though the pregnancy rate per cycle may be as high as 30 per cent. ZIFT is also very expensive as it involves multiple procedures.

The zygotes are transferred on day 1 after fertilization using laparoscopic techniques under general anaesthetic (for more information on laparoscopy see Chapter 7, Medical and surgical treatment). The developing zygotes are passed through a tube into the fallopian tubes. Currently two zygotes can be transferred, which then must travel through the tubes to the uterus to implant to develop into a viable pregnancy. If the embryos are transferred into the tubes on day 2 after fertilization, the technique is termed tubal embryo transfer (TET); it may give the advantage of being able to pick bigger and hopefully healthier embryos. ZIFT has a high rate of multiple pregnancy.

Pre-implantation genetic diagnosis (PGD)

Many of us are carriers of genetic diseases that, if we have children with another carrier of the same disease, we could pass on to our children who would be affected. These genes are called recessive genes and are hidden within our cells without causing us any adverse effects. For example, one in 25 of us is a carrier for cystic fibrosis without having any evidence of the disease in ourselves. Alternatively you may know that you have a disease that you could pass on to your children.

Prior to pre-implantation genetic diagnosis the only methods to detect whether or not the unborn foetus was affected by a genetic disease were either to wait until the foetus was born and test it, or wait and see if it developed the illness; or to have prenatal testing. Prenatal testing involves either chorionic villous sampling (CVS) at 10–14 weeks gestation or amniocentesis at 16–18 weeks of pregnancy, both of which carry a risk of miscarriage. If the foetus is affected by the disease in question you have a choice as to whether or not you wish to continue the pregnancy. This decision may be made harder by the fact that you may be three to five months pregnant at the time of diagnosis.

PGD involves testing embryos before they are transferred to the uterus. Only non-affected embryos are transferred back so you can be reassured that your foetus will not be affected. It is used in couples where there is a high risk of any pregnancy being affected by a disease for which we know the causative gene and where to find it on the chromosomes, for example, couples who have had a previously affected child, are known to be carriers or are affected by a genetic disease, or who have had recurrent miscarriages known to be caused by a genetic problem. Diseases for which embryos can be screened include cystic fibrosis, Down's syndrome, Tay-Sachs disease and sickle cell anaemia.

Pre-implantation screening (PGS) is similar to PGD but there is no specific disease that is being looked for. It can be used in those over 35, those with recurrent miscarriage or failed IVF cycles, or those at increased risk of chromosome abnormalities. The embryos are screened to check if they have the correct number of chromosomes (aneuploidy screening).

> I had been through the process before. I had a child, Jenny with Rett's syndrome, a genetic disorder that affects only girls. I love her to pieces but her life is hard, she will never be able to talk or feed herself, never mind support herself, and regularly has fits. It is both for us as parents and for the child that we went for PGD as we felt supporting two affected children would have been almost impossible. Why bring another child into this world to suffer? Although Jenny laughs, she also cries, is she happy? I don't know. I want to have a child that I know will be happy, that I know will be able to cope in this world when we are no longer here to help. It is not that we don't value Jenny, of course we do, we just

> don't want to have another suffering child, and that is why we are using PGD. (Betty, 36)

The procedure involves IVF, even if the couple is fertile. After fertilization, the developing embryos are incubated as normal. On day 3, when the embryos are at the six to eight cell stage, one or two cells are removed through a small hole made in the shell of the embryo. Each cell contains all the genes and so it does not matter which cells are removed; the cell that is taken is then tested for the genetic disease. The results should be available within 24 hours so embryo transfer takes place on day 4 or 5 after fertilization. In this way the embryos can be divided into those that are affected and those that are unaffected, and only unaffected embryos will then be transferred back in the hope of developing into a pregnancy.

Risks

PGD carries the same risks as for all IVF treatments. It is also possible that in removing a cell, the embryo can become damaged resulting in foetal abnormality or embryo death.

Chances of success

Once the unaffected embryos are transferred back into the uterus, the chances of success are that of a conventional IVF cycle. The chances of obtaining unaffected embryos are dependent on the number of eggs collected and then fertilized and the genetics of the disease in question.

Assisted hatching

Assisted hatching aims to help the embryo implant into the lining of the womb. During the very early stages of development, the embryo is surrounded by a thick layer of protective proteins called the zona pellucida. When the embryo reaches the uterus, it has to 'hatch' out of this protective layer in order to implant into the endometrium. It is thought that some embryos, perhaps those from older eggs, have a zona that is very thick and the embryos have difficulty in hatching, so implantation cannot occur. The aim of assisted hatching is to help the embryo shed its protective lining and implant into the womb.

Assisted hatching may be suitable for couples who have not been successful with conventional IVF cycles, for older women or for women with hormone results suggesting a diminished ovarian reserve.

The procedure involves all the same stages as IVF. However, before transferring the embryo back on the third or fourth day after fertilization, a small hole is made in the zona pellucida. The embryo is then washed and transferred back into the uterus on the same day.

Risks

These are the same as those associated with IVF. There is also an increased chance with assisted hatching of having identical twins, as the action of creating a hole in the outer shell of the embryo may cause the embryo to split. If the embryo is damaged during the procedure, there is a risk of foetal deformities and even embryo death.

> I am not sure what would be worse – transferring embryos back and then not getting pregnant, or having assisted hatching and then losing two of my three embryos to the procedure, leaving me with only one on which to pin my hopes. Will I get pregnant because of or in spite of the assisted hatching? (Sophie, 43)

Chances of success

Some studies suggest that the rates of pregnancy with assisted hatching IVF are higher than with IVF alone. However, at present there is little reproducible evidence to suggest that assisted hatching increases the chances of pregnancy or the rate of live births.

Frozen embryo cycles

If you have chosen to freeze embryos (cryopreservation) from previous cycles these can be used in future IVF cycles. You will not need to take the medication to induce ovulation if you are using cryopreserved embryos. You will have regular ultrasounds to monitor the thickness of the lining of the womb. At the optimum time in your natural cycle, about two to three days after ovulation, when the endometrium is thick and ready for implantation, the embryos will be thawed and transferred into your uterus in the same procedure as used in IVF.

Risks

At present it is not known what, if any, the effects of cryopreservation may be on the embryo.

Chances of success

About two-thirds to 70 per cent of the embryos will survive the freezing and thawing process. After transfer the success rate is similar to that in IVF.

Ethical issues

The processes involved in assisted reproduction may bring up ethical or religious issues or concerns. As with many of the questions involved in the treatment of subfertility, there are no correct answers, only how you feel and what is right for you. You may feel that you want to carry out more research into certain issues or may want to involve a religious or spiritual adviser to help you make decisions. For each person or couple the issues causing concern may be different or occur at different points in your journey. Many of the issues mentioned below have been the subjects of court cases and appeals and there may be legal requirements, such as those for the storage of embryos or sex selection. Your opinions may affect how your treatment is carried out. Clinics must offer counselling to couples undergoing subfertility treatment; if you felt comfortable it may be a useful time to talk about some of your feelings about these issues.

The list of topics for discussion below could never be complete; as technology changes and medicine advances more and more, other issues may arise. Some of the ideas mentioned are controversial. My aim is not to offend, but to suggest some opinions that you may not have considered, or may disagree with, in order to further your own discussions.

Some issues you may like to discuss could include:

- Where do you feel life begins? Does life begin in each sperm or egg or does it begin when the sperm fertilizes the egg to form a zygote, or when it is an embryo, or foetus or only when the baby is born and is physically separated from its mother?
- Legally in the UK an embryo under 24 weeks of pregnancy does not have any rights. A foetus born after 24 weeks gestation has the right to resuscitation and medical treatment; this legal right only begins after the baby is born, as before then it is not considered alive. How do you feel about this?
- If you feel that life begins with sperm and eggs – how do you feel about masturbation needed to produce sperm samples? Do you feel that all eggs retrieved should be fertilized, irrespective of their maturity?
- How do you feel about the embryos themselves? Currently in the UK, in most cases only two embryos are transferred back into the woman, though this may decrease to only one embryo. If there are surplus embryos, what do you feel should happen to them? Would you like them to be frozen (cryopreservation) or should they be

destroyed? What options does your clinic offer you? If you decide to freeze extra embryos, how long do you want to keep them, and what will you do, and how will you feel, when you decide you don't want them any more?

- The doctors decide which embryos to put back on the basis of which they think are the most healthy – how do you feel about this? Is this saying that the others weren't good enough?
- If you are having ICSI – how do you feel about a doctor choosing which sperm with which to inject your eggs? The particular sperm they use will decide half of the genes of your future child; different sperm would create a different child. What about the rest of the sperm – what should happen to it?
- If you are having PGD – is this saying that those with a disability or certain disease are not as worthy of life as others?
- Is it reasonable to use PGD to create a child in order to try and save the life of another, for example a child who would be able to give marrow for a bone marrow transplant?
- How would you feel if PGD were taken further and one could decide the sex of one's child and other physical or mental characteristics? Would we end up with a 'superior race' of tall, intelligent and athletic people?
- If you freeze your sperm, eggs or embryos – who has rights to them if you split up or if one partner dies? What would those rights mean – rights to have a child with someone even if they did not want to? Is this the same as a form of rape?
- If you are using donor sperm, eggs or embryos, or are using a surrogate, what do you think is acceptable to know about your donor/surrogate? What rights, if any, to the child should the donor or surrogate have? What rights should the child have to find out about the donor/surrogate?
- If you are using donors or surrogates – should they be paid or is this the same as selling a child? Some clinics offer free/cut price treatment to women who donate eggs. What do you feel about that?
- How old is too old to have a baby?
- Does everyone have the right to have a child, no matter what the cost?

9

Donors, surrogacy, fostering and adoption

It may be that the treatments described in the previous chapter may not work or may not be suitable in your situation. In this case it may be appropriate to involve other people in order to create your family. This can involve using donors or surrogates. A further alternative is adoption in which you take parental responsibility for a child that is not genetically your own. Each of these situations brings up many emotional and ethical issues and counselling is mandatory. The situations described below are closely regulated by the law.

Donors

Donor eggs, sperm or embryos can be used in subfertility treatment. Some of the topics mentioned in counselling sessions may include:

- What will you tell your child about how they were conceived?
- How do you feel about accepting half or all of your child's genes from someone you don't know?
- If you are using a known donor, how much input do you feel they will have in your child's upbringing?
- How would you feel if your child attempts to contact the donor? Or if they made contact and the donor accepted/rejected them?
- How do you feel about your child potentially having other brothers and sisters that they do not know?

The legal issues around donation

> I thought it mattered that my child looked like me, talked like me, had my mannerisms and physical characteristics. I wanted to do all the father–son things like going to the football and having people say he was the spit of me. Letting go of that was difficult. My wife didn't really get it, after all, she was still going to be related to the child, genetically, and I would never be. Years on, I've realized that my boy does talk like me, he does have my man-

> nerisms and in a way does look like me, in the way that he does things. I guess it is not just about genetics. (Ken, 47)

Legally, the mother of a child is the woman who gives birth to it and her partner the father, irrespective of whether donor sperm, eggs or embryos are used. The law states that any child born as a result of a donor (after April 2005) has the right to find out information about the donor. This information is held by the HFEA and includes information about physical characteristics, ethnic group, other children they may have, medical history and information such as a message from the donor to the child. If the child is planning to start a serious relationship he or she can also check whether or not he or she is related to the potential partner. The child can also apply for contact information such as the donor's last known address.

Donors can be known to you (such as family or friends) or anonymous. Donors undergo screening: medical and family histories, their chromosomes are checked for abnormalities and they are screened for diseases such as hepatitis and HIV. Sperm donors must be between 18 and 40 and egg donors below 35.

Sperm donation

Semen is examined for quality and quantity of sperm and then frozen for six months. At the end of this time a further HIV test is carried out as you can be infected with HIV but have no evidence of it for a period of time. You may be able to choose donors that have similar physical characteristics to yourself.

> If you would have asked me when I started fertility treatment whether or not I would consider using donor sperm I probably would have said no. Then again, had you asked me ten years ago if I would have IVF I probably would have also said no. My husband has a 'moderate reduction in sperm count, but significant numbers of abnormal forms'. Initially, rather hopefully looking back on it, we tried IUI, then IVF and then ICSI, but I didn't become pregnant. After two IVF cycles and three of ICSI we just felt that we couldn't do it any more, and I felt that I couldn't keep putting my body through so many procedures. So we went for donor insemination and here I am, with our child. Admittedly the thought of someone else's sperm inside me was weird but this is definitely our baby. (Sarah, 33)

If you are not using known donors, your clinic may be able to put you in touch with a sperm bank or put you on the waiting list for eggs or embryos. You can advertise for an egg donor (but a potential donor cannot advertise her services), or you can get involved in an egg sharing scheme if you are able to pay for both your treatment and that of your donor. Donors are not paid, though they may have their expenses covered. If you are using donors from abroad it is important to check their selection and screening processes to ensure that the donations are healthy and safe. Donors can change their minds about the use of their donation but only until they are used. Once insemination or fertilization has occurred, donors no longer have rights to their sperm/eggs or embryos. The donors themselves also undergo counselling.

Donor sperm can be used if you have a poor sperm count, are worried about passing on an infection or genetic disease, or for single parents or same sex partnerships. The sperm can be used in artificial insemination or IVF depending on whether there are also female factors involved. Donor insemination may be cheaper and less invasive than ICSI techniques and therefore for some couples may be preferable. If there is enough sperm, you could use sperm from the same donor to have more than one child so your children will be entirely genetically related. One donor can be used by up to ten different people.

Donor eggs

Donor eggs can be used if you are not producing eggs, or producing only a few eggs, if there is a risk of passing on a genetic disease, or if you have had failed IVF cycles or recurrent miscarriages. You take medications to time your cycle with that of the donor so that your endometrium is thick and ready for implantation at the time of transfer. The donor undergoes superovulation and eggs are collected and used in IVF, ICSI or GIFT.

Donated eggs are currently not frozen, as the effect of freezing on egg quality is not known, so they are only tested once; therefore there is a very small risk of passing on HIV. From the stage of embryo transfer, the process is the same as for women using their own eggs. The success rates of donor egg IVF are higher than with conventional IVF, about 25–40 per cent per cycle, perhaps as eggs from women under 35 are of better quality.

Donor embryos

Donor eggs and sperm can be used in the same treatment or donor embryos can be used. Donated embryos are frozen for six months for infection screening. At the time in your cycle when you are ready for implantation, the donor embryos (which have been unfrozen) are transferred into you as with conventional IVF. Donated embryos are those from other couples who have finished their families or have decided to stop treatment and have surplus frozen embryos, and have given their written consent to donate them to other people.

> Using donor embryos always seemed a rather wonderful and uplifting idea. I knew that this couple could have children, they had completed their family (three kids!) and had some spare frozen embryos. So, if they could have children with these embryos so could we! I liked the fact that I would still go through pregnancy and labour, that I could breastfeed my child. They gave me the greatest gift imaginable, my baby. (Katie, 41)

Surrogacy

Surrogacy involves a woman carrying and then giving birth to a child for another woman. It can be used if you cannot carry a pregnancy. One or both of you can be genetically related to the child. Surrogacy is controlled by the law; it is advisable that you seek the advice of a solicitor during this process. Some topics discussed in counselling may include:

- Is your surrogate a family member, or friend? If so, how much input do you think, and do they think, they should have in your child's upbringing?
- What will you tell the child?
- Will you keep in touch with the surrogate?
- How do you feel about another woman going through the process of pregnancy and birth with 'your' child?
- When will the child be handed over? At the birth? Would you allow the surrogate to breastfeed the child?
- Do you trust your surrogate? For example, to stay healthy during the pregnancy, to make appropriate health-related decisions during the pregnancy and birth both for herself and for the baby? Do you want antenatal screening for various diseases, and does she agree? Do you trust her not to change her mind?

The legal process of surrogacy

You, as the person or couple wishing to bring up the child, are called the 'commissioner'. The woman who becomes pregnant is called the 'surrogate'. Before conception itself, an agreement is made in which the surrogate agrees to give the child to the commissioner. Surrogacy can be described as when one woman acts as the incubator for another. There are two types of surrogacy, depending on whose gametes are used:

- *Full or traditional surrogacy* The surrogate uses her own eggs and the sperm either of the commissioner or a donor, to become pregnant. Artificial insemination or IVF can be used. In this situation, the surrogate is the genetic mother of any child produced.
- *Partial or gestational or host surrogacy* The commissioner's eggs and sperm, or donor sperm, or donor eggs and commissioner's or donor sperm are used in IVF in order for the surrogate to become pregnant.

> They weren't my eggs though they were my husband's sperm, and it wasn't my body that grew and nurtured the embryo. But it is my baby. (Eleanor, 39)

You have to find a surrogate yourself, either from friends or family or someone previously unknown to you. It is illegal to advertise for a surrogate. There are various surrogacy support groups; talking to others and finding out how they found surrogates may be helpful. Some potential surrogates may contact surrogacy support groups in the hope of meeting commissioning couples/intended parents. The law states that only married couples who are resident in the UK can be involved in surrogacy; unfortunately this excludes same sex couples who have undergone a civil ceremony and single parents (though in the UK you can adopt a child).

> I had to have my womb and ovaries removed when I was in my early 20s. I was lucky in that my sister had always said that she would carry my child for me. My husband was very supportive and although there were a few initial jokes and weird silences about the fact that essentially she would be making a baby with my husband (though without the sex), we came to an agreement. I liked the thought that this baby would be as genetically close to me as possible.
>
> We went to infertility counselling, surrogacy counselling and family counselling, sometimes on my own, with my husband or the four of us together. I think some of my family thought it was odd and definitely I worried that she wouldn't be able to let go. It must have been hard for her, we were there when my baby girl was born, they put her on my tummy and that was it, I knew she was mine. My sister didn't really get involved with my daughter

for a few months, we had agreed that would be best and now she is simply the best auntie. I will tell my baby about how special her auntie is, that she gave me the opportunity to be a mummy. I will never stop being grateful. (Anne, 34)

You cannot pay your surrogate a salary. You can pay 'reasonable' expenses, including life insurance or critical illness cover in case she falls ill related to the process of conception or the pregnancy, loss of earnings, travel expenses and the cost of medical treatment.

Who are the legal parents?

The woman that gives birth to a child is its legal parent, and her name is put on the birth certificate. In Scotland, if the commissioner's sperm is used, his name is on the birth certificate as the legal father; outside Scotland this is not possible. If the surrogate puts her partner on the birth certificate, he is the legal father, unless he writes a letter saying that he did not agree to the pregnancy, in which case the commissioning man, or intended father, can be put on the birth certificate. In all situations the child can be registered with its intended parents' surname. If the intended father has his name on the birth certificate, he is also the legal father. If not, the intended father can apply for a 'Parental Responsibility Agreement', which gives you equal rights to the baby with the surrogate.

Six weeks after the birth the commissioning couple can apply for a parental order or adopt the child. To apply for a parental order, one of the commissioning couple needs to be genetically related to the child – that is, they must have provided either the egg or the sperm. The child must be living with you. You and your surrogate will be visited by a court representative to check among other things that the surrogate has given consent and was not salaried. You can apply for a parental order up to six months after the baby is born. If a parental order is given the surrogate gives up all rights to the child. You then get a new birth certificate with your names on as mother and father.

If neither of you are genetically related to the baby you must then apply (in conjunction with an adoption agency) to adopt the child.

Up to the point that a parental order or adoption is obtained, the surrogate can refuse to give up the child. Whether or not the child is genetically related to her, the law states that as the legal mother, she has the right to keep the child. Fortunately, this is rare, but possible, and for the commissioning couple is devastating.

Adoption

Adoption is a legal process in which you are given full parental rights and responsibilities of a child that is not genetically your own. Questions to ask yourself include:

- How do I feel about caring for a child that is not my own?
- Does this mean that we have stopped trying for our own child?
- How do we feel about not knowing much about the child's origins or family history?
- How would we feel about not adopting a baby, but a child?
- How do we feel about adopting a child of a different race from our own?
- What would we tell the child? The current advice is that children should be told of their origins.
- What would we tell our families?
- How would we feel if our child wants to find his/her birth parents?

> What is a parent? When we realized that it just wasn't working for us, that we were never going to actually produce a child, I looked it up in the dictionary. According to them, a parent is someone who brings a child into the world. Well, I think they are wrong, a parent is someone who brings up a child, who cares for it, nurtures it, supports it, loves it. The genetics have never mattered, I am a parent. (Jonathan, 36)

You can be married, single, co-habiting, heterosexual or in a same sex relationship to adopt. Adoption is carried out through an adoption agency. The process is rigorous and involves multiple assessments of yourself and your ability to care for a child; it takes at least six months. Although you have to be over 21 to adopt a child, there is no upper age limit; as long as you are healthy and able to care for a child, you should be considered. There may be a very long wait to adopt a child under one year of age; more older children are available. Children put up for adoption are not all given up at birth, and many have been in foster homes prior to adoption. You can take the equivalent of maternity leave after adopting a child.

It is also possible to adopt from outside the UK, though this has to be approved by social services and the Home Office. If you are adopting a child from abroad, he or she has to be living with you for a year before you can apply for an adoption order.

Depending on the age of the child, the process is a gradual one in which the child is introduced to you and then visits your home for increasing periods of time, all in close association with the adoption agency and social services. In order to apply for an adoption order, the child has to have lived with you for at least 13 weeks.

The earliest point at which a baby can move in with you is at six weeks old. A court representative checks with the birth parents that they understand the procedure and that they give up their rights to their child. If they do not, but the child is still suitable for adoption, for example if social services have removed a child, the court still has the power to grant an adoption order, though this may take a longer period of time. If appropriate, the birth parents may communicate with the child via the adoption agency.

> I knew that there were children out there who needed me, and who needed love. We were desperate for children, and in their own ways my children were desperate for us, for the love and support that we give them. We have always told them that they have other parents who love them, but couldn't look after them and so they gave them to us. It was never a big revelation, just something that my kids have always known. If they choose to go looking for their birth parents, I hope that I will be secure enough in the knowledge of how they feel about me, that I am there to help with homework, to nurse them when they are sick, that I will be the one in the memories of their childhood. After all, I am their mother, and they are my children. (Tilly, 41)

Fostering

Fostering is similar to adoption. However, you do not have sole parental responsibility for the child, as this is shared with the local authority. This can be a temporary or long-term agreement. Foster parents are paid allowances by the local authority to cover the costs of caring for the child. Children can be fostered if they or their families are having problems and need short-term or permanent respite.

Although many of the children available for fostering and adoption are healthy, there is a group of children that may have physical and/or emotional difficulties. In this case, you should be offered counselling and support from a social worker.

10

Emotional issues

The process of trying to get pregnant is a stressful and emotional time even if you do not have any fertility problems. For couples with subfertility the pressures and stresses of conception are heightened. You experience many emotions during your journey, ranging from hope, fear, anger and joy to uncertainty and anxiety. You may also be concerned about some of the ethical issues brought up by assisted conception techniques. Having someone to talk to, be it your partner, friends or a counsellor, can be invaluable. If you do get pregnant, your emotions can become even more complex, including increased anxiety. Finally there is perhaps the hardest decision of all, the decision to stop treatment and accept a life without children.

Counselling

We often counsel each other when we talk to our family and friends about our lives, situations, feelings and any difficulties we may be having. We talk, they listen, sometimes they offer advice and other times they just sympathize. When it is their turn, we do the same for them. In broad terms, counsellors, who may be experts in fertility or relationship issues, do a similar job. The main difference between a counsellor and your normal confidantes is that the counsellor does not already know you. He or she is objective, does not already have an opinion of you, and will not get bored of you or judge you. Whatever you say in a counselling session is confidential.

Clinics must offer you implications counselling before treatment. Going to counselling is only mandatory if you are using donors or surrogates as they may bring about more complicated emotions. Bear in mind that counselling may not be included in the price of treatment. Support counselling can be with a single counsellor or within a support group. You could have sessions every week, a short burst of sessions or just occasionally when you feel you need it.

Going to counselling does not mean that you are going mad or not coping. It is an opportunity to talk about how you feel, and discuss various options, perhaps again and again, in a way that your friends may not tolerate. It can help you understand how you are feeling, and make some potentially difficult decisions. Your counsellor is there to support you, whatever your choices, and help you find ways to support and talk to each other and to cope with problems. Counsellors do not necessarily give advice or tell you what you should do (even if sometimes you want someone to do exactly that); they simply help you to come to your own decisions by examining your emotions. You can see a counsellor alone or with your partner or other family members.

> All I ever thought about was a baby. I would almost become paralysed with sadness in the supermarket when I passed the nappy aisle. Friends who had babies made me feel empty, and I felt I couldn't truly be happy for them when I was so bitterly jealous. My counsellor helped me realize that it wasn't my friends' faults that I needed fertility treatment! I realized that although they have children, perhaps they could imagine what I was feeling even more than my friends without children, as they know what I am missing. (Catherine, 38)

No topic is taboo with your counsellor. This may include subjects that you may find difficult to bring up with your partner, such as wanting to stop treatment, or difficulties with sex. There could be issues which are causing tension between you as a couple, for example a previous sexually transmitted disease. Don't feel that a subject or a feeling is stupid – if you feel it, then it is valid.

Many situations outside those of procedures and treatments can become unbearable. These can include close friends or family becoming pregnant, baby showers, or once the baby is born; family parties where relatives say things like 'No sign of a baby yet then?' or look at your tummy in a way you feel is disapproving. Telling people may not result in the support you had hoped for; some people cannot handle the emotions of others, and may brush you off or patronize you. A boss who is unsympathetic to your need to have time off for appointments, or even a parent or sibling who in trying to be supportive is actually being overpowering and claustrophobic, can all cause intolerable stress. A counsellor may help you deal with some of these emotions.

> I am in my early 30s and come from a large and close family. We all get together often and there are lots of babies and children running around. I began to find them intolerable. I felt like a barren woman and that the babies were there to taunt me. The continual barrage of questions about whether I was trying, if I was trying was there a problem, what was I doing, did I know this

> doctor, that someone had found a new treatment on the net, etc., etc., etc.! At the time I found it unbearable. I didn't appreciate that everyone cared about us and were trying to help. I used to make jokes about how great it was to be able to have a cream sofa and not worry about little dirty handprints. With the support of my husband I stopped making jokes and starting telling people that Tom and I were having problems conceiving and that while we appreciated their help and advice we were finding it all a little confusing and overpowering to have so many opinions. We then chose just to tell our parents what we were doing. It was amazing, the emphasis changed from questioning us to helping us – everything from offering us lifts to appointments to things like taking us out for dinner. (Yvonne, 35)

Support groups can play many of the same roles as a counsellor, often in a more informal setting. Knowing that other people are experiencing the same emotions and situations that you are experiencing can be empowering and help you feel that you are not alone. You could also make new friends.

Your partner

The person who is often your biggest support – and sometimes your biggest concern – is your partner. After all, you are trying to make a baby, together. Feelings of guilt are common, and it is very easy to transfer a feeling of guilt into one of blame. You may have differing views about treatment and some of the ethical questions that may arise. It cannot be stressed enough that you have to keep talking and keep listening to each other.

> I try and talk to my wife, but every time I do, she just brushes me off saying something like, we will get pregnant, we will succeed as we want it so much. She says that she needs to stay positive, and that she can't listen to me telling her that it might not work in case it brings her down. But I need her to know that I am scared, scared that it won't work and that if it fails I won't be able to support her. Most of the time it is fine, I believe we will have a child, but when I get doubtful I want someone to say that I am right, that perhaps it won't work, but that there is a chance that it will and we have to hold on to that, and to hope for the best, prepare for the worst. The more she says it will work, the more I worry it won't. (Tim, 37)

Try and ensure that your partner feels that you are giving him or her your full attention when he or she is talking about feelings. Try not to respond with negatives such as 'You're wrong' but with non-inflammatory statements such as 'I see why you feel like that, but I feel differently because …' Your partner's feelings are just as valid as your own, whether or not you feel they are logical.

Just as important as talking about your fertility is not talking about your fertility. Your life is not just about having a baby, though sometimes it may feel that way. You probably have many other things in your lives, and after all you have each other. Make time to talk about other things, go out, have fun and try to be as relaxed as you can be. Hopefully this will help make the bad times easier, as you and your partner will be a strong unit.

> All we would talk about was having a baby, our whole lives were driven by it. We made new friends at our support group and gradually stopped seeing our old friends who either did or did not have babies – either way we felt that they would not understand. So we went out with our new friends and talked shop. After a few months, my husband said that he was beginning to forget that we had ever not been trying for a baby, that we had ever been happy on our own. It shocked me and made me realize just how one track minded we had become. I made the effort to contact our friends and we started going out more, being together and having fun. The mood in the house lightened and became more hopeful. (Esme, 31)

> For us, it was about taking control back over our lives. Not letting us be defined by our infertility. Going out, stopping worrying if we had sex on the third day instead of alternate days, forgetting to take my temperature once in a while, having the odd glass of wine. It was empowering, we were back in control and it felt good. (Pat, 37)

Deciding when to stop, and moving on

Deciding to end your treatment can be one of the hardest decisions you ever make. You have probably spent a long time wanting and trying to have a child. You have put yourself through physical, emotional and sometimes financial stress in order to do so, and yet it has not worked. It can be hard to stop trying, harder to stop wanting.

> Whenever I have wanted something I put my mind to it and worked out a way to achieve it – getting a good job, getting on the

> property ladder, finding a relationship, and then having a baby. No matter what I threw at the problem, I could not resolve it. My body just wouldn't listen to my mind, it was so frustrating. Why wasn't it working? (Melissa, 38)

Potential reasons why treatment has not worked include that no eggs are collected, no eggs fertilize or develop or they don't implant. No matter what the reason, the actual problem may not actually matter: the end point is still that you have not got pregnant. There are many implications:

> We had always planned to have a family. We talked about our hopes for children from very early on in our relationship. I worry that if I can't give my partner the children that he wants, he will find someone who will. (Donna, 41)

Treatment for subfertility is exhausting on many levels – physical, emotional and financial. The decision to stop may be made for any reason. Even broaching the subject of stopping treatment can be scary and you may feel that your partner may be disappointed. As in every stage of your journey, keep talking; involving a counsellor may be helpful.

> I didn't want to be the one to say, enough. My partner appeared to be as keen for the next cycle of IVF as she was for the first, and I was worried she would think I was giving up on her. When I finally did mention that I was finding it difficult, she cried with relief. She had been feeling the same way but hadn't wanted to disappoint me. (Jack, 39)

Telling people may be difficult; they may not understand, or may push you to keep trying. In the end, though, you have to do what is best for you. No one else can tell you what is right or wrong for you.

> Telling my mum was hard. She was so desperate for me to have the same joy that I brought to her. She kept on telling me to keep trying, but it is my body and only I can decide what is best for me. (Amy, 42)

> I felt like I lost the support of my support group. Before, we always joked that we were failures together – now I felt that I had failed at failing. (Betty, 39)

Ending fertility treatment does not necessarily mean ending your decision to have a child. Other options such as fostering or adoption may still be available. Bear in mind too that if you do decide that you are not going to try for a family, your decision does not have to be for ever.

If you change your minds, then you can always get back into the system. Deciding to stop treatment is not the same as giving up, but about moving on.

> I was just relieved. It had taken up so much of our lives for so long. Now we can do something else. (Max, 44)

> I mourned, initially every time I had a period, then every time IVF didn't work. Finally I grieved for what I couldn't have. Now I can move on. (Robin, 40)

While for some people stopping is not an acceptable option, for others it can act as closure on a difficult period of their life, allowing them to move on to new things.

> Occasionally I still look longingly at my sister's children, but most of the time I focus on my new role: cool, fun auntie. I've got my life back. (Clara, 39)

> I spent 16 years striving to become pregnant, praying I would become pregnant. During that whole period of my life I had always felt that something was missing in our lives and that it would only be by having children that we would be complete. So deciding to stop felt like I was accepting that feeling of emptiness, I honestly thought I would never truly be happy. It has been most pleasingly surprising to discover I was wrong – our lives are now more full than ever, with exciting new challenges and achievements. (Janice, 44)

> I was unhappy, now I am content. (Sharon, 37)

You've got pregnant!

First, congratulations!

Your clinic may offer you an early pregnancy scan. If you want your antenatal care on the NHS, see your GP who will arrange your care from 12 weeks of pregnancy. After having difficulties in becoming pregnant, the emotions when you get pregnant can be overwhelming. You may not be overjoyed all of the time and this is okay – it can be difficult to be in the greatest of spirits if you have morning sickness or breast soreness. Even if you feel well physically, the emotional upheaval of actually being pregnant may be stressful. You may be concerned about miscarriage or multiple births. Your clinic may offer counselling in early pregnancy.

11

Complementary treatments and relaxation techniques

Complementary medicine is not alternative but can be used alongside traditional medicine. The techniques often take a holistic approach, looking at the body as a whole, not just at your fertility. It is important that you inform both your traditional doctor and any complementary therapist of any treatment or medication that you may be taking as they may interact with other medicines. Even if you do not feel that a treatment is helping with your fertility, it may have the benefit of being relaxing. The list below is not exhaustive.

Acupuncture

Acupuncture is part of traditional Chinese medicine. The belief is that diseases occur due to imbalances of Qi (energy) in the body. Imbalances occur for many reasons including hereditary factors and diet. Acupuncture involves inserting fine needles into the energy pathways (meridians) in the body to correct the imbalances, thereby restoring the balance of yin and yang in the body. Sterile single-use needles should be used. Studies have shown that acupuncture can be used beneficially in the treatment of subfertility.

Aromatherapy

Aromatherapy involves the use of plant essences and their scents, either by inhaling or by massage. The basic principle is that the plants can be used to stimulate the body's immune system to help the body heal itself. For example, clary sage and rose oils are thought to aid fertility, and are also said to be aphrodisiacs.

Ayurvedic medicine

Sometimes called Indian traditional medicine, this is based on the philosophy that the body is formed of elements such as water and earth to form three 'doshas': wind, phlegm and bile. Each dosha has a function, and an imbalance of these can cause disease. Treatment can involve a combination of herbs, dietary advice, massage, yoga and relaxation techniques.

Bach Flower Remedies

Bach Flower Remedies use plants or flowers taken in a tincture. The belief is that in order to be healthy in body, you need to be healthy in mind and that negative emotional states can lead to disease. Tinctures are taken for certain feelings: for hopelessness – gorse, for feelings of despair – sweet chestnut. Rescue remedy is a combination of five different plants and can be used in stressful situations. Remedies can be obtained from many high street shops and pharmacies.

Herbalism

Herbalism uses the healing properties of plants. Herbalism is used in Chinese medicine, Ayurvedic medicine and medical herbalism. Medical herbalism aims to avoid the side effects of synthetic drugs. For example, agnus castus (chasteberry) can be used to treat female subfertility.

Homeopathy

Homeopathy aims to help the body heal itself by correcting any imbalances. Homeopathy uses minute amounts of diluted organic substances to treat conditions. Your treatment will be made specifically for your combination of symptoms. Note that any symptoms may initially worsen during treatment; this is thought to show that the treatment is working.

Reflexology

The theory behind reflexology is that the body's organs and energy can be mapped on to the feet and can therefore be manipulated via pressure and massage to the feet to unblock energy and purge the body of waste products.

Reiki

Reiki is a form of healing. It involves the practitioner gently placing their hands over parts of the body to either give or remove energy to ensure balance within the body.

Shiatsu

Shiatsu is a form of massage (often done through a layer of clothing) in which the practitioner uses their hands to place pressure on certain parts of your body to unblock trapped energy and restore balance to the body.

Traditional Chinese medicine

The theory behind Chinese medicine is that the opposing energies of yin and yang in the body must be balanced, as imbalances lead to disease. The energies can be rebalanced using a combination of herbs, acupuncture, acupressure, massage, exercise and lifestyle advice. Chinese herbs include dong quai (angelica) and Hachimijiogan (a blend of herbs) for female subfertility and cornus officinalis to improve sperm quality.

Relaxation techniques

The following techniques may be used to help you relax and decrease stress. Try the techniques sitting in a comfortable position, or lying down with your eyes closed. You may initially find these techniques difficult; after all, you have a lot to think about. However, it may be worth persevering to see if they really can help you relax. With time, you may be able to use these techniques at stressful points during your day.

Breathing techniques

Focusing on your breathing can bring a sense of calm. The breathing techniques can be used alone or with any of the other techniques described.

- Try and focus solely on your breathing.
- Breathe in through your nose for a count of three. Try to be aware of using your whole chest and feeling your chest open fully.
- Pause at the top for a count of three (or one if you feel breathless)

and then exhale for a count of three. Feel the air leave your lungs either through your nose or a gently open mouth. You could try saying a word in your head as you exhale such as 'relax' or 'gently'.
- Then repeat.
- Try and think of your breathing as an oval shape, one side is the inhale and the other the exhale. They are a connected and continuous cycle.
- Continue for about ten minutes or as long as you need.

As you get used to the technique you may not need to count your breathing, but if you get distracted return to the counting. If you have said a word during your exhale, try saying it at a stressful time to try and remind you of the relaxed feeling you had during the exercise.

Visualization or imagery techniques

During your breathing, imagine that you are in a place where you are happy and relaxed. Try and use all your senses: feel the warmth of the sun or a cool breeze, smell the grass, hear the sea. Now think of a place or situation that makes you stressed or anxious, such as the hospital, and then imagine it shrinking. Again try and use all your senses, for example the sound of the people becoming quieter and quieter until you can't hear them. Shrink this 'bad place' so you can pick it up, then either imagine throwing it away or imagine it continuing to shrink until it is the size of a stamp, then a pin head and then it disappears.

Alternatively you could imagine your 'bad place' and try and change it in your head, fill it with light, warmth, colour and feelings of happiness so that it can no longer harm you. Also try imagining that you are something strong, like a house or an ancient tree. Visualize your body as strong, like the tree with strong roots or the house with its foundations that anchor you. When you feel stressed remember the feeling of being anchored to help give you strength.

Physical relaxation techniques

- Focus on each muscle group or part of your body in turn, tense it and then relax. For example, start with your feet or calves, tense the muscles tightly and then focus on them relaxing. Feel and imagine them warm and heavy and sinking into the floor or bed. Continue with each muscle in turn from the feet up, including the muscles in your shoulders, neck, jaw and head until you are relaxed.
- Try focusing on relaxing your body every time you exhale.
- Saying something like 'I am relaxed, my legs/arms, etc. feel warm and heavy' may help.

- Imagine a wave of relaxation, perhaps like a shower or waterfall coming from above your head and passing over your body, relaxing each part of your body in turn.
- Imagine that the floor or bed you are lying on is a calming colour such as blue or green. See the colour rising from the floor through your feet and up your body; as the colour fills your body you relax.
- Yoga techniques and stretching can be used.

Diaries

Write a diary and include all the bad thoughts and ideas that pop into your head as well as all the difficult situations you have experienced. For some people, writing down their feelings may be enough to help let them go. Others may need to go through the diary and assess each emotion: Why did you feel that way? What could you change to make you feel better? Perhaps imagine what you would say if a friend told you what they were feeling as you wrote in your diary – how would you advise them?

Affirmations

Creating positive affirmations for every negative emotion can also be helpful. For example, if you wrote:

> I felt frustrated about having to wait 20 minutes for my appointment.

You could write something like:

> I am grateful that my doctor will give me extra time if I need it and I am happy that today I feel I don't need the extra time because I feel calm and prepared.

Or if you wrote:

> I feel helpless.

Try writing:

> I feel it will happen for me – it may take time, but I will achieve my desires.

12

Future developments

Medicine and technology are quickly changing and developing. Research is continually being carried out into the causes, treatment and prevention of subfertility. Many of the subjects discussed in scientific journals, on the internet and in newspapers are not yet available in clinics. The list below is not exhaustive; as we find out more, there will be more treatments available.

Some of the treatments below are offered in some clinics but not all. They are often controversial as the majority of doctors feel there is not enough evidence about the risks and benefits of the treatment to feel confident about offering the treatment. However, some medical professionals, and indeed you, may feel that even a low chance is worth trying. Not all of these treatments are regulated by the HFEA.

Egg cryopreservation

It is currently possible to freeze eggs, though the success rates of IVF when using frozen eggs compared to fresh eggs is low. Further advances in this field may enable eggs to be frozen, for example before cancer treatment, and then used successfully in IVF.

In vitro maturation (IVM)

In vitro maturation is a form of IVF which does not involve the superovulation stage. During the early part of the woman's cycle, very low doses of drugs are given and immature eggs are then removed from the ovaries; these are then matured in the laboratory with FSH. After about 24–48 hours they are thought to be mature enough for fertilization, and the embryos are then transferred back into the woman as with conventional IVF. Initial trials show pregnancy rates of approximately 30 per cent per cycle, without the use of high levels of potentially harmful medications.

Uterus transplant

Womb transplants could be used for women who do not have wombs. They could be transplanted for the amount of time needed to become pregnant and carry a child before being removed again, preventing the need for long-term use of immunosuppressant medications to stop rejection.

Ovary transplant

Ovary transplants could be used for those who have undergone a premature menopause. Only a small section of an ovary would need to be transplanted. Currently there has been a successful ovarian transplant in the USA using identical twins. Ovary transplants could also be 'auto-transplants', that is a transplant from yourself. It may be possible to remove and freeze a section of healthy ovary before undergoing, for example, chemotherapy or radiotherapy. This may then be transplanted back once therapy is complete.

Pre-implantation embryo screening

Currently two embryos are transferred back into the woman in IVF, and this may be decreased to only one embryo in the future. Techniques may be developed to enable doctors to pick the healthiest embryos, and therefore those most likely to implant and develop into a pregnancy, to transfer back. Currently it is possible to screen for common abnormalities in chromosome number, and this screening may be expanded.

Treatment of immunological subfertility

In some circumstances IVF is successful up until the stage of implantation; it may be that the woman's immune system then attacks the embryo and prevents it implanting, or attacks it once it has been implanted. Some clinics offer medications such as immunoglobulins or steroids in the hope of preventing this occurring.

And finally . . .

I remember wondering as a child whether I was a wanted baby or a 'mistake'. It wasn't that I didn't feel loved or wanted, it was just that when I found out about the facts of life and things like contraception I began to wonder if I had been planned. My child will never need to wonder whether or not she was wanted, she will know that she was. I tell her that mummy had to have lots of tests and visits to the doctor, that I knew that she would be so special that she was worth having injections and procedures for. She will know that we wanted her so much we would have done almost anything to have her. She will know that she was truly wanted, and is truly loved. (Penny, 32)

Useful addresses

ACeBabes
No office as the charity is run by its members on a voluntary basis, but for privacy or an urgent enquiry write to:
PO Box 6979
Derby
DE1 9HY
Tel.: 0845 838 1593 (sometimes an answerphone but all calls are treated in confidence; if possible, however, contact by email)
Website: www.acebabes.co.uk
Email: enquiries@acebabes.co.uk

Offers support: on pregnancy after fertility treatment; decisions such as using donors; what to do with embryos; trying for further children; what to tell children.

Adoption and Fostering Information Line (AFIL)
204 Stockport Road
Altrincham WA15 7UA
Freephone: 0800 783 4086
Website: www.adoption.org.uk

Provides information and support for those considering adoption.

Adoption UK
46 The Green
South Bar Street
Banbury
Oxon OX16 9AB
Tel.: 01295 752240
Website: www.adoptionuk.org

Provides information and support for those considering adoption.

British Association for Adoption and Fostering (BAAF)
Saffron House
6–10 Kirby Street
London EC1N 8TS
Tel.: 020 7421 2600
Website: www.baaf.org.uk

Provides information and support for those considering fostering or adopting, and the website gives details of regional offices.

British Association for Sexual and Relationship Therapy (BASRT)
Tel.: 020 8543 2707
Website: www.basrt.org.uk

A charity for sexual, couple and relationship therapy.

British Infertility Counselling Association (BICA)
Tel.: 01744 750660
Website: http://74.220.205.213/bica/

Founded in 1988 as a membership charitable organization for professional infertility counsellors. Promotes and gives information about finding a subfertility counsellor.

Childlessness Overcome Through Surrogacy (COTS)
Lairg
Sutherland IV27 4EF
Tel.: 0844 414 0181 (local rate); 01549 402777
Website: www.surrogacy.org.uk

Support group for those using surrogacy.

Daisy Network
PO Box 183
Rossendale BB4 6WZ
Website: www.daisynetwork.org.uk

Support and information membership network for women with premature menopause. A not-for-profit organization with no office or paid staff. If writing for information rather than accessing the website, please enclose s.a.e.

Donor Conception Network (DC Network)
PO Box 7471
Nottingham NG3 6ZR
Tel.: 020 8245 4369
Website: www.donor-conception-network.org

Self-help support network for those using donor gametes or embryos and their children.

Endometriosis UK (formerly **National Endometriosis Society**)
50 Westminster Palace Gardens
Artillery Row
London SW1P 1RR
Tel.: 0808 808 2227
Website: www.endo.org.uk

Fostering Network (formerly **National Foster Care Association)**
87 Blackfriars Road
London SE1 8HA
Tel.: 020 7620 6400
Website: www.fostering.net

Provides information and support for those considering fostering. There are also offices in Belfast, Cardiff and Glasgow.

Human Fertilization and Embryology Authority (HFEA)
21 Bloomsbury Street
London WC1B 3HF
Tel.: 020 7291 8200
Website: www.hfea.gov.uk

Information for patients and their supporters on all aspects of subfertility and its treatment.

Infertility Network UK (INUK)
Charter House
43 St Leonard's Road
Bexhill on Sea
East Sussex TN40 1JA
Tel.: 08701 188088
Website: www.infertilitynetworkuk.com

Offers support and advice for those with subfertility and infertility. It also runs the More to Life grouping for couples who wish to stop treatment.

Institute for Complementary Medicine
PO Box 194
London SE16 7QZ
Tel.: 020 7237 5165
Website: www.i-c-m.org.uk

Provides information on complementary medicines and how to obtain them.

Miscarriage Association
C/o Clayton Hospital
Northgate
Wakefield
West Yorkshire WF1 3JS
Tel.: 01924 200 799
Website: www.miscarriageassociation.org.uk

Gives support and information for women and couples who have had a miscarriage.

Multiple Births Foundation
Hammersmith House, Level 4
Queen Charlotte's and Chelsea Hospital
Du Cane Road
London W12 0HS
Tel.: 020 8383 3519
Website: www.multiplebirths.org.uk

National Childbirth Trust (NCT)
Alexandra House
Oldham Terrace
Acton
London W3 6NH
Enquiry Line: 0870 444 8707
Website: www.nct.org.uk

Provides information regarding pregnancy and parenthood.

National Gamete Donation Trust (NGDT)
PO Box 2121
Gloucester GL19 4WT
Tel.: 0845 226 9193
Website: www.ngdt.co.uk

For those considering becoming egg or sperm donors, health professionals, and those requiring treatment with donor eggs or sperm.

Relate
Herbert Gray College
Little Church Street
Rugby CV21 3AP
Tel: 0845 456 1310
Website: www.relate.org.uk

Offers relationship and sexual support and counselling; there are Relate branches all over the UK.

Surrogacy UK
PO Box 24
Newent
Gloucestershire GL18 1YS
Tel.: 01531 821889
Website: www.surrogacyuk.org

Support group for couples using surrogacy.

UK Donorlink
31 Moor Road
Headingley
Leeds LS6 4BG
Tel.: 0113 278 3217
Website: www.ukdonorlink.org.uk

A support network and a voluntary register for those conceived from donors.

Verity
Unit AS20.01
Aberdeen Centre
22–24 Highbury Grove
London N5 2EA
Website: www.verity-pcos.org.uk

A support group for women with polycystic ovary syndrome. No office telephone yet; if funding allows it is hoped that a helpline can be set up.

Index